How to Help Clients Get the Most Out of Rational Emotive Behaviour Therapy

This book aims to assist therapists in helping their clients decide if Rational Emotive Behaviour Therapy (REBT) is for them and, if so, how to get the most out of the model.

It does not seek to equip therapists with the particular REBT skills presented in training courses and skills-oriented books but rather strives to help therapists and their clients to be aware of and deal productively with more general issues that pertain to the effective practice of REBT. Topics covered include:

- Helping clients decide if REBT is for them.
- Helping clients prepare for their REBT sessions.
- Helping clients understand the process of change in REBT.
- Helping clients apply what they learn from REBT sessions.
- Helping clients become their own REBT therapist.

This book is designed for all REBT therapists, whether experienced or in training.

Windy Dryden is in part-time clinical and consultative practice and is an international authority on REBT. He has worked in psychotherapy for more than 45 years and is the author and editor of over 285 books.

How to Help Clients Get the Most Out of Rational Emotive Behaviour Therapy

A Practitioner's Guide

Windy Dryden

Routledge
Taylor & Francis Group
LONDON AND NEW YORK

First published 2026
by Routledge
4 Park Square, Milton Park, Abingdon, Oxon OX14 4RN

and by Routledge
605 Third Avenue, New York, NY 10158

Routledge is an imprint of the Taylor & Francis Group, an informa business

British Library Cataloguing-in-Publication Data
A catalogue record for this book is available from the British Library

ISBN: 9781032796413 (hbk)
ISBN: 9781032796031 (pbk)
ISBN: 9781003493150 (ebk)

DOI: 10.4324/9781003493150

Typeset in Times New Roman
by Newgen Publishing UK

I dedicate this book to the following people who have shown enduring commitment to me and to my work: Anna Albright, Wouter Backx, Rhena Branch, Trecia Cohen, Kristene Doyle, Louise Dryden, Nicola Hurton, Avy Joseph, Walter Matweychuk, Martin Noble, Arthur Still, Peter Trower, John Viterito, Matthew Walters, Rob Willson and John Wilson.

Contents

Introduction

I have written this book for you whether you are a novice REBT therapist, a more experienced REBT practitioner or an REBT therapist in training. My goal is to assist you in helping your clients decide if REBT is for them and, if so, in helping them to get the most out of REBT. You may wish to know that I have written a companion book for clients in which I deal with similar issues that you will find in this book, but from a client perspective. It might be useful to suggest to your clients that they consult the companion client book so that you are conjointly aware of the salient issues that occur at relevant points during the REBT process and can use the book as a vehicle for discussion, if helpful.

As you will see, what this book does *not* seek to do is equip you with particular REBT skills. You will have acquired such skills on your training course and from skills-oriented books and other materials. The companion client book does not seek to equip clients with REBT skills either. What both books do is help you and your client be aware of and deal productively with more general issues that pertain to the effective practice of REBT and not with the approach-specific skills that may be found in the burgeoning REBT literature written for both therapists and clients. As such, taken together, these books are designed to help your clients get the most out of REBT.

DOI: 10.4324/9781003493150-1

This book is intended to be a practical guide and not an academic one. As such it will contain no references so that you can keep your focus on matters of practice.

Windy Dryden
London, Eastbourne

Chapter 1

Help Your Clients Decide if REBT Is for Them

How is it that people who have just approached you for help have decided to consult an REBT therapist? Have they made a definite commitment to do this or are they still thinking about it? How much do they know about REBT? Have they actively sought out an REBT therapist on their own or were they recommended to do so? These are some of the questions that may come into your mind as prospective clients make contact with you or enter your consulting room.[1] Indeed, these are some of the questions that I do ask people who come to see me either to consult me as an REBT practitioner or to seek my help in assisting them to determine which approach to therapy is best suited to them. As you won't know the answers to these questions, let me start by dealing with the issue of how you can best help your prospective clients decide if REBT is for them in a more general way.

Common Factors That Span Therapy Approaches

In the field of psychotherapy and counselling it is recognized that different approaches have both common factors (i.e. common to all therapeutic approaches) and specific factors (i.e. specific to the particular approach under consideration). The main common factors include:

• The development and maintenance of an effective working alliance between you and your clients.

DOI: 10.4324/9781003493150-2

- The provision of a safe space in which you can help your clients discuss whatever is important to them.
- The mobilization of hope whereby your clients come to see that they can effectively address their concerns.
- Your clients experiencing you, as therapist, as someone who is genuine with them, understands them and accepts them.

As I have said, these factors are common to all approaches to therapy and are not specific to REBT.

While I have entitled this chapter 'Help Your Clients Decide if REBT Is for Them', when it comes to the presence or absence of these common factors, I suggest that your focus be more on helping your prospective clients to decide whether or not you are the right *person* for them to consult rather than on whether or not REBT is right for them. Thus, you may be as a therapist technically proficient in REBT, but if a prospective client does not feel safe talking to you about what really matters to them, they are right to have doubts about you as their therapist. It follows from this that your principal general therapeutic goals at the outset are to:

- Develop an effective working alliance between you and your clients.
- Provide a safe space in which your clients feel able to discuss whatever is important to them.
- Help your clients to see that they can effectively address their concerns.
- Show your clients that you are genuine with them, can understand them from their frame of reference and accept them warts and all.
- Establish a communication forum between you and your clients where you can both talk freely about your mutual experiences of therapy. I call this establishing a meta-therapy dialogue.

While it is unrealistic for you as a therapist to score top marks on all these points, you should aim to score highly enough for your prospective clients to consider working with you over time. If you score poorly on all these points with a particular client, then, in all probability, you will not be able to help them much despite your proficiency in REBT. However, you should take your work with this client to supervision as a matter of priority at the first sign that you have a general problem with working with the person. I will discuss this issue more fully in Chapter 7.

If you score highly on all but one or two points, then you should again seek supervisory help, but therapy with the client is probably still viable. In the client companion to this book, I recommend, in this situation, that your client should consider discussing their feelings with you on the points where you do not score highly. If they do, it is very important that you listen to them non-defensively and initiate a dialogue to address their concerns. If they do not do so, but you sense that they do have concerns about your interaction in some areas, raise this possibility with them gently to help them express themself. Showing your client that you have noticed that they may have concerns about you as a therapist and that you genuinely wish to hear what they are so you can deal with them is often therapeutic in itself. If you deal defensively with your client on this matter, then they may leave therapy. If you experience defensiveness with your clients, once again discuss them in supervision. Having made this point, don't forget that therapists are human too and you may have the odd off day.

I will address the importance of discussing matters to do with therapy with your clients more fully later in this book.

REBT's Main Specific Factors

When your prospective clients are coming to a decision concerning REBT's suitability for them, it is important for them to understand some of the therapy's main features. REBT is, in fact, a particular approach within a larger psychotherapy tradition known as Cognitive Behaviour Therapy (CBT), and it may be that your client is seeking you out because you are a CBT therapist and not an REBT therapist. Having said that, let me outline some of REBT's main specific factors that you may wish to inform your prospective clients about.

Some REBT therapists will send prospective clients a brief description of REBT so that they can see if it is an approach that they may be interested in. An example of such a description is found in Appendix 1.

Help Your Clients Understand That REBT Focuses on the Way People Act and Think in the Context of Their Emotions and the Situations in Which They Experience These Emotions

Remind your clients that REBT stands for 'Rational Emotive Behaviour Therapy', but as this approach falls under the CBT tradition, they should expect that therapy will focus on behaviour and cognition.

Focus on Behaviour

I suggest that you start with behaviour, as this is the easiest of the two terms for clients to grasp. Prime your clients to expect that as an REBT therapist you will focus a lot on the ways in which they behave, particularly in situations in which they experience their problem(s). However, show them that you are also interested to understand what may be termed their 'action tendencies'. Explain that these describe situations in which clients feel an urge to act in a certain way but don't actually do so. Show them that such action tendencies are particularly valuable in helping you to discover their hard-to-identify emotions (such as envy and hurt). Helping clients understand the difference between an action tendency and an overt behaviour may help them see that they don't have to act on their action tendencies, which is particularly important with problems of anger and self-discipline.

It is also useful to help your clients understand that the behavioural focus in REBT is particularly linked to an understanding of their goals and values. Thus, they should expect that you will enquire about the extent to which their problem-related behaviour helps them to meet their goals and the extent to which it is consistent with their personally held values. Consequently, prime your clients to expect that you will encourage them to act in ways that help them to achieve their goals and are consistent with their values, as well as helping them to identify, reflect on and deal with obstacles to the execution of such behaviour.

If your clients experience anxiety, in particular, show them that a particular behavioural focus that you are likely to take is on their use of safety behaviours. Help them to understand that such behaviours are employed by clients to keep them safe from threat but in ways that *may* serve to maintain their problems. Remember that REBT and CBT practice is strongly underpinned by research; while studies in the past showed the negative effects of such safety behaviours, more recent studies have shown that such behaviours may be useful in encouraging your clients to face their fears. Here, as elsewhere, effective REBT therapists keep abreast of the research literature and modify their practice accordingly.

Focus on Thinking

In REBT, help your clients to understand that you will be focusing on thinking that has a bearing on how they feel and act. While there are different types of thinking, emphasize that you will be focusing mainly on the rigid and extreme attitudes that in REBT we say lie at the base of your clients' emotional and behavioural problems. In addition, help them see that you will also be working with the inferences that they make in problem-related situations but that you will often encourage them to assume temporarily that their inferences are correct so that you can help them pinpoint the rigid and extreme attitudes that from an REBT perspective explain the presence of their problems. Be ready to provide them with examples so this principle is very clear to them.

Here, as elsewhere, it is important that you are to be transparent in explaining your position on these issues to your clients, that you ensure that your points have been understood, that you give your clients an opportunity to raise any concerns that they have concerning your explanation and that you correct, with respect, any misconceptions that your clients reveal.

Help Your Clients Understand That REBT Focuses on How They Unwittingly Maintain Their Problems Rather Than on How These Problems Originally Began. Consequently, They Should Realize That REBT Focuses on What They Can Do Now to Address Their Problems

Some clients come to REBT not knowing anything about this approach and may have internalized a common view about therapy: that they are expected to talk about their past. Other clients may come to REBT thinking that you will not be interested in their past at all. The truth, of course, is somewhere in the middle. Help both sets of clients understand that they may talk about whatever it is they are bothered about, be it their past, their present or their future. Having said this, you need to help them see that in REBT, in general, we tend not to believe that helping clients to understand the past roots of their present problems will be curative in the long term without their doing something about these problems in the present. Of course, you need to stress that their relevant past experiences may have contributed to their current problems, but having said that, these past experiences do not account fully for these problems. A common way of explaining this is by pointing out that if 100 people all experienced exactly the same adversities in the past as your client, not all of them would have developed the same problems as the client. Some may have developed other problems and others would not have developed problems at all. Rather, it is important that you help your clients understand that it is the attitudes that they developed from these experiences and still hold currently that largely accounts for their problems, together with the behaviours that stem from and are associated with these attitudes.

You might wish to use the problem of jealousy as an example here. Help your clients understand that if they have such a problem, it may well be the case that they felt jealous of one of their siblings as a child. However, explain that this insight will not help them if they continue to act in jealous ways in the present (e.g. by preventing their partner from doing things, checking on their whereabouts). Such behaviour will reinforce and strengthen the rigid and extreme attitudes that underpin their jealous feelings and will nullify any effect that insight into the possible roots of their problem might have. As a result, explain that unless you help your clients to deal with the ways in which they currently, but unwittingly, maintain their problems, then it is unlikely that they will gain much long-term benefit from therapy.

Encourage Your Clients to Understand That REBT Focuses on Helping Them to Put into Practice Between Sessions What They Learn in Sessions

It is important that you help your clients understand, in the first place, that it is unlikely that they will derive any benefit from REBT unless they learn something in therapy sessions. However, it is perhaps more important that you help them see that such learning is likely to be academic and thus of limited value to them unless they put this learning into practice between therapy sessions. Consequently, help your clients appreciate that in REBT, one of your major tasks as an REBT therapist is to negotiate with them ways of implementing their session-derived insights into relevant situations in their everyday lives. They should understand that the extent to which you negotiate suitable tasks with them and the extent to which they effectively implement these tasks will help determine how much they will get from REBT. I often tell my clients that when I am asked whether REBT is helpful, my answer is: Yes, if clients use it; no, if they don't! I will discuss in Chapter 6 the issue of helping clients to apply what they learn.

It Is Useful to Outline to Your Clients That REBT Focuses on Helping Them to Become Their Own REBT Therapist

While all approaches to counselling and psychotherapy have as an aim clients learning how to help themselves in the future after therapy has ended, it is important to explain that as an REBT therapist you will strive to implement this aim in specific ways with your clients, perhaps more specifically than therapists from other therapeutic orientations. Explain to your clients that, if appropriate, you will do this by teaching them REBT self-help skills throughout the therapy process.

Inform them that you may well use an REBT-related framework to teach them how to assess their rigid and extreme attitudes, disturbed feelings and unconstructive behaviour in problem-related episodes and how to respond productively to these situations. Say that you will then encourage them to use this framework for themselves between sessions and that you will help them to refine their developing skills in subsequent sessions when they report back on how they implemented their skills. Given this emphasis on helping clients to become their own REBT therapist, tell them that it is likely that you will give them increasing responsibility to help themselves as therapy progresses. Explain that you will do this by gradually fading your own active contribution to the process over time, later becoming more of a consultant, giving your clients feedback on their developing self-helping skills rather than continuing to take an active lead as you did at the beginning of therapy.

Because REBT emphasizes teaching clients self-help skills, there are a number of REBT-oriented workbooks available that can be used as an adjunct to therapy. You may suggest to your clients incorporating such a workbook into their therapy.

While some clients value using such workbooks, others find them too formulaic and would prefer not to use them.

Also, if you are a flexible REBT therapist, you will be mindful of the fact that while REBT does emphasize the teaching of self-help skills as an integral part of the therapy, some clients do not want to learn these skills in such a deliberate manner. You should aim to adjust REBT accordingly. I will discuss the issue of helping your clients to become their own REBT therapist more fully in Chapter 8.

In this chapter, I have outlined some of REBT's distinctive features for you to explain to clients, both prospective and actual. I have also argued that you need to stress to clients that REBT values explicitness and that you will make clear to them how you are likely to use REBT to understand and deal with their problems. As a result, it should be easier for clients to judge whether or not REBT is right for them or whether it would be better for them to consult a therapist who practises a different CBT approach to REBT or a non-CBT approach. If some are still in doubt, suggest to them a brief 'trial period' of REBT where they can experience this approach to therapy for themselves as a way of judging whether or not they wish to make a firm commitment to becoming an REBT client.

If clients have decided that REBT is right for them and want to work with you, you will need to make a number of practical agreements with them to ensure that therapy gets off on the right foot. This will be the subject of the next chapter.

Note

1   In this book, by consulting room I mean a space where you may see your clients face-to-face or online.

Chapter 2

Make Practical Agreements with Your Clients

Therapy, of whatever type, works better if the two involved parties, namely you and your client, agree on a number of important points. These points can be placed in one of two realms: the practical realm of REBT and the therapeutic realm of REBT.

The practical realm of REBT involves such matters as your fee, if one is charged, and how it is to be paid; how frequently you will meet your clients; how many sessions you will have with clients; and what your cancellation policy is. If you work in a clinic, then there may well be additional practical issues to be discussed and agreed to. I will deal with such practical agreements in this chapter.

The therapeutic realm of REBT involves such matters as how you and your client see their problems and what their respective goals are with respect to these problems. It also involves understanding what steps you are both going to take to address your client's problems and help them to achieve their goals and the commitment they are prepared to make with respect to carrying out these steps. I will deal with such therapeutic agreements in the next chapter.

While the distinction between the practical and therapeutic realms of REBT is somewhat arbitrary – after all, how you and your client negotiate on the practical issues may either be therapeutic or non-therapeutic – it is a useful way of separating out issues concerning why they have come for therapy and what they want to achieve (i.e. the therapeutic realm) and issues that

DOI: 10.4324/9781003493150-3

are designed to grease the wheels for both of you (i.e. the practical realm) as you help your client strive to achieve their goals. So here are some of the practical agreements you will need to make with your clients.

The Length of Therapy Sessions

One of the practical aspects of therapy that you should make clear at the outset is the length of therapy sessions. Actually, it is likely that when most clients think of therapy 'sessions', they think that the 'therapeutic hour' lasts a full hour rather than 50 minutes. They don't know that the tradition of the 50-minute therapeutic hour has come about to reflect the fact that therapists need to take a short break between sessions for several reasons, most typically to write notes, clear their head, go to the toilet or make and/or take phone calls. If you operate a 50-minute-hour practice, then you should make this clear to your clients. Otherwise, they may think that your sessions last for 60 minutes and may consider that they have been short-changed if you stop sessions after 50 minutes without explanation. Sometimes, therapy sessions with clients may be shorter or longer, and if any changes are made to an established and agreed arrangement with respect to the length of therapy sessions, then this needs to be fully discussed, understood and agreed to by both of you. I suggest that if any changes are made to an established session length, you agree with your clients, in advance, pro rata changes to any fees that are being charged (see the next section).

Your Fee

If you work as an REBT therapist in a National Health Service (NHS) clinic or facility or in an organization that does not levy a fee, then what I have to say does not concern you, although if this is the case, it is very likely that the number of sessions you can agree to have with your client will be limited (see the section, 'The Total Number of REBT Sessions', later in the chapter). However, if it is the case that you do levy a fee, then it is very important that your clients understand what this fee is. I have known clients who have not enquired about their therapist's fees and have had quite a shock when they received the latter's invoice because the therapist, in these cases, had not told the clients what their fees were. So please do make clear what your fee is as early as possible, whether or not your clients ask for it. I suggest that you do this on initial enquiry to save time. If your fees are out of a client's financial reach, it is useful to tell them whether you have a sliding fee scale. If not, or if the reduced fee is still out of your client's range, then it is useful to inform them whether you have a colleague whose fees are within their range. Ask your clients explicitly, then, how much they are prepared to pay.

Your clients may well be thinking that how much they can afford per therapy session will be based on how many sessions they will need. However, they need to understand that at the very outset you cannot tell them how many sessions they may need until you have carried out a thorough assessment of their problems.

When you and your clients have agreed to a fee, you need to explain to them whether the fee (or part of it) will be levied if you contact and discuss matters with them between sessions or if a fee will be charged for other matters. For example, I once saw a client for individual REBT who, at the same time, was having couples therapy with a different therapist. The client had to be hospitalized but requested a couples therapy session while she was in hospital. The couples therapist came to the hospital and duly conducted the session. To my client's surprise and consternation, the therapist billed the couple for three hours as opposed to the usual one-hour charge for the session. When questioned, the therapist told the couple that he was billing them for the one-hour session and the two hours that he gave up to travel to and from the hospital to carry out the session.

The point that I wish to make here does not concern the rights and wrongs of charging for two hours of travel time but concerns the fact that the therapist did not make clear that he was going to do this in advance of agreeing to carry out the hospital-based therapy session. Also, the client couple could have asked if there was going to be an additional charge, as the therapist would have to make the journey out of his professional time. This failure to make an agreement about the additional charge, which I argue is in the practical realm of therapy, had quite an adverse effect on the therapeutic relationship and it took quite a while for the therapist to regain the couple's trust in him.

To avoid such misunderstandings, follow a simple rule: explain to your clients everything they need to know about your position on fees so that they can decide whether or not they wish to proceed with therapy on the basis of this position or whether they wish to question it or suggest modifications to it. You should listen respectfully to such suggested modifications and discuss the issues that these raise before deciding whether or not to agree to them.

Your Cancellation Policy

When you contract with your clients, and if you do levy a fee, then it is important that you explain to your clients what your cancellation policy is. Once they understand this, they may wish to suggest amendments based on their unique circumstances. This should lead to a discussion and hopefully to a mutually agreed policy. Possible ambiguities of the terms of the policy should be highlighted by one or both parties and clarified. For example, I have a 48-hour cancellation policy, which, as I point out to prospective clients, is different from one specifying two days. Thus, if a client and I have scheduled for, say, 11am on Wednesday and they wish to cancel it without paying my fee, then they need to inform me of that by 11am on the Monday before. If they cancel their appointment at 12 noon on Monday, they will be charged, since they has not given me the full 48 hours' notice.

You may or may not charge a fee if a client cancels a session without giving full notice if they become ill or a member of their family becomes ill, for example. Again, it is important that you are clear with your clients about the exceptions you are prepared to make concerning fee payment when a client has not given full notice.

Some therapists apply their cancellation policy to themselves, while others don't. For example, if I have to cancel a client's session and I have not given them 48 hours' notice, then their next scheduled session is provided free of charge. Again, you should ideally make this explicit to your clients if you follow my lead.

The Total Number of REBT Sessions

It is very likely that when prospective clients are thinking about consulting you as an REBT therapist, they are wondering how many sessions they are likely to need. However, while this is a reasonable question for them to ask you from their perspective, it is important for you to explain that the number of sessions they will need cannot be validly determined by you when they first contact you, as all they have probably done is to give you very rudimentary information about themselves and their problems. You need to explain to these prospective clients that you can only responsibly answer this question after you have met with them and carried out a full assessment of their problems and what they want to achieve from therapy. Having said that, here is what I say to prospective clients:

The length of therapy depends on how many problems you have, what you want to achieve with respect to these problems, how chronic your problems are and how hard you work in therapy. So, if you have a few problems that are acute in nature, are prepared to work hard to address these problems in between therapy sessions and to work towards achievable, specific goals, then therapy is likely to be short-term in nature. However, if you have a large number of problems that are chronic in nature, you think that change will occur in therapy sessions rather than by what you do between sessions and your goals are vague, then therapy is likely to be longer term.

You may wish to develop something similar to tell your clients who want to know something about how many sessions they are likely to need before you have carried out a full problem and goal assessment.

The Frequency of REBT Sessions

Normally, your clients will see you once a week until they make progress, and then sessions are likely to be spaced out more. This is because a major goal of REBT is for your clients to become their own therapist, as I mentioned in Chapter 1 and as I will discuss more fully in Chapter 8. As your clients learn the skills of REBT, you will urge them to take increasing responsibility for applying these skills in their lives, and the increasing spacing out of therapy sessions encourages them to do that. You should explain this to your clients so they understand it when you suggest increasing the frequency between sessions.

There may be times when you see a client more than once a week. This may reflect the complexity of their problems or that they are going through a crisis; both of these situations indicate that they need more therapeutic input than weekly sessions. However, even under these conditions, you should encourage them to take responsibility for dealing with these issues as far as they are able and suggest reducing the frequency of sessions when they are ready to do so. This readiness will be assessed by you and your client together.

Confidentiality

Your clients may think that the contact between you and them is completely confidential, but in reality, this is unlikely to be the case. Here is a list of situations where you may reveal information about your clients or take action without their permission:

- When mandated to do so by the courts.
- To protect a client's well-being when they are not able or willing to do so.
- To protect the well-being of others when your client poses a threat to them without your client taking steps to protect these others.
- If a client steadfastly refuses to pay your fees and you take legal action to be paid.

You may have additional exceptions to complete confidentiality, and if so, you should inform your clients about these in addition to those listed above. This latter point is the main one that I wish to stress. One of the ethical principles that counselling and psychotherapy is based on is *informed consent.* From your clients' perspective, this means that you need to clearly inform them about something before they can properly consent to it. Because one of the features of REBT is its explicitness, you should, ideally, make explicit all the exceptions to complete confidentiality.

The Form of the Contract

So far, in this chapter, I have focused on the practical agreements that you need to make with your clients if you are to help them to get the most out of REBT. While the important point is that these agreements should be made, you and your clients need to determine together the form that they will take. Thus, such agreements may be made informally or formally.

An informally made agreement tends to be verbal, and as such it is open to misinterpretation and misunderstanding. Thus, earlier I mentioned that I have a 48-hour cancellation policy. If I explain what this means verbally, my clients may not understand what I have said or forget the nature of the policy. This may lead to problems later when a particular client fails to give the stated notice and questions why they must pay for the cancelled session.

A formally made agreement tends to be written and may even be signed by both parties. While such an agreement is not open to misinterpretation or misunderstanding, it may well put off some clients who complain that it is too businesslike and indicates that you do not trust them. In Appendix 2, you will find an example of a formal agreement.

My point here is to state the importance of you and your clients agreeing on the form of the contract you have decided to make, in light of the fact that both the informal and formal approaches to contracting have their advantages and disadvantages.

Having dealt with the practical agreements that you will need to make with your clients as an REBT therapist, I now, in the next chapter, consider the therapeutic agreements you will need to make with them.

Chapter 3

Make Therapeutic Agreements with Your Clients

In the previous chapter, I discussed a number of practical agreements that it is important for you to make with your clients if your working relationship with them is going to get off on the right foot and stay that way. However, most of these practical agreements are common to most, if not all, approaches to therapy and are certainly not unique to REBT. In this chapter, I am going to focus on the therapeutic agreements you need to make with your clients that do pertain to REBT and concern why they have, in the main, come for therapy: to address their emotional problems and get on with the business of living.

While clients who are seeing non-REBT therapists will make similar agreements, I will concentrate here on agreements that typify REBT. As I have already mentioned, one of the features of REBT that characterizes this therapeutic approach is its emphasis on explicitness. As a therapist, you will spell out what you mean about a number of important issues, as we shall see. If you are not being clear about something, then you should encourage your clients to tell you so. If you are not prepared to tell your clients something, then you should explain the reason(s) why not. The distinct advantage of therapist explicitness is that it enables your clients to understand where you, as their therapist, are coming from and to agree or disagree with the explicitly expressed points you have made.

In this chapter, I will discuss the nature of the therapeutic agreements that you need to make with your clients, facilitated as these agreements are by your explicit style of communication. Later in this chapter, I will discuss the importance of helping your clients to speak up if there is anything they don't understand about what you are saying, if they disagree with anything that you say or if they find anything that you say or do unhelpful.

The Nature of Therapeutic Agreements

In this section I will discuss six different types of therapeutic agreements you need to make with your clients. While your agreement on some points may be more explicit than on others, for REBT to be fully effective you need to have clear agreement on all six points.

Agreements about Your Clients' Problem(s)

Your clients have probably come to REBT because they have one or more emotional or behavioural problems for which they are seeking help. It is important that you listen carefully to these problems and communicate that you understand how they see these problems from their frame of reference and acknowledge that they do, in fact, want to address these problems. Later, you will offer them an REBT-based understanding of these problems, but at the outset, it is important that you agree with them concerning which problems they wish to address. You may introduce your clients to the idea of a *problem list*, on which they put, in writing, what problems they want to cover in therapy. Explain to them that this list is not set in stone and that they may add to it or subtract from it over the course of therapy.

Also, you need to explain to your clients that, generally, only problems that are within their control to tackle should be on the list and that those that are outside their control should not be included. Thus, if one of your clients is very angry with his (in this case) partner's untidiness around the house and yells at her and argues that his problem is his partner's untidiness, then you need to explain that because this behaviour is under his partner's control rather than his own, you cannot legitimately place a change in this behaviour on the therapy agenda. You need to help him to see that what is under his control are his feelings (unhealthy anger) and his behaviour (yelling). As these are unlikely to help him effectively address his partner's untidiness with her (in this case), you need to invite him to regard his feelings and behaviour as problematic in this context and thus to put his *response to her untidiness* on the problem list rather than the untidiness itself.

Generally, only emotional and/or behavioural problems should be put on the problem list and not practical problems, and you should explain why to your clients. Thus, if a client is experiencing financial problems in their life, then explain that this, on its own, is not a matter that can be directly dealt with by REBT. Rather, your client needs to consult a debt counsellor or financial adviser for such practical problems. However, your client may also have emotional problems over these practical financial matters, and these emotional problems can be tackled by REBT and may, with your client's assent, be placed on their problem list.

Agreements about Your Clients' Goals

For every problem that a client seeks help for, it is useful for you both to have as clear an idea as you can about what your client wants to achieve. So, you need to take a goal-oriented focus together with a problem-oriented focus.

I usually explain the importance of goals like this to my clients:

Imagine that you go to a railway terminus and say to the person selling tickets, 'I don't want to go to Brighton'. This person will either be at a loss as to what to do or will sell you a ticket for anywhere that is not Brighton. In either case, you are likely to be unhappy with the result. In the same way as expressing clearly where you want to go to a train ticket seller, doing the same thing with me, your REBT therapist, will aid both of us to collaborate on working towards achieving your therapeutic goals.

To help your clients with goal setting, you may wish to make use of the acronym 'SMART' to indicate the criteria for clearly formulated goals. Explain to your clients that:

• *S* stands for 'specific'. Help your clients to understand that the more specific they can be about their goals, the more they will be able to see how to achieve them. Explain that goals such as 'I want to be happy', while laudable, are very vague and as such will be difficult for your clients to achieve. On the other hand, the goal 'I want to deal with the prospect of criticism with healthy concern rather than anxiety and approach people who I think may criticize me rather than avoid them' is a clearly expressed goal, and its specificity will help this client to achieve it.
• *M* stands for 'measurable'. Help your clients to understand that the more they can measure progress towards their goals, the more likely it is that they will persist with taking steps to achieve them. For example, if a client comes with the goal 'I want to tidy my house', show them that this is difficult to measure, whereas the goal 'I want to spend one hour a day tidying my house' is measurable and your client can track their progress towards achieving it.
• *A* stands for 'attainable'. Help your clients to understand the importance of setting goals that can actually be achieved by them. Thus, if a client states the goal 'I want to be free from anxiety', help them to see that this is probably unachievable, whereas the goal 'I want to respond to feeling anxious by working towards feeling healthy concern' is attainable.

- *R* stands for 'realistic'. Your clients may set a goal that is attainable (e.g. 'I want to exercise in the gym for an hour a day'), but it may not be realistic for them to achieve it. Thus, one of your clients may live very far from a gym, and their work and family commitments may be too onerous for them to achieve this goal. While it is attainable in the sense that they have the ability to do it, it is not realistic in that they cannot find the time to do it. By contrast, 'exercising for twenty minutes a day by running around the nearby park' may be both attainable and realistic. Thus, explain to clients the difference between goals that are attainable and realistic and goals that are attainable but unrealistic, and help them to set the former rather than the latter.
- *T* stands for 'time-bound'. Help your clients to understand that it is important for them to set a time frame for achieving their goals. Show them that if they do not do this, they may be tempted to keep postponing working towards achieving them. Invite your clients to compare the time-unbound goal 'I want to write my paper' with the more time-bound goal 'I want to write my paper by the end of this month'. The latter imbues the goal-setter with a greater sense of urgency than the former. Also, help your clients to see that while it is important to give themselves a specific time frame to achieve their goal, they need to ensure that this frame is realistic and gives them some margin for error.

While it is important for you to keep the concept of SMART goals in mind when working with your clients, do not impose it on them in a slavish manner. As I stress throughout this book, competent REBT therapists are flexible, and, as such, while you may think that encouraging your clients to develop SMART goals is the best way to help them get the most out of REBT, you also need to recognize that some may not find the development of such goals helpful, or some of their problems may not lend themselves to such an approach to goal formulation. In such cases, you need to help clients to formulate goals that make sense to both of you. You may need to engage in some negotiation over this point, but a jointly agreed goal is more likely to be achieved by your clients than one that is either imposed on them or about which you as therapist have serious reservations. Before leaving the topic of goals, I want to make one other important point. Help your clients to understand that they are more likely to achieve them if they are prepared to commit themselves to achieving them and to accept the sacrifices that goal pursuit inevitably involves. I use the following vignette to press home this point with some clients:

> Two friends, John and Jack, struggle with procrastination and are falling behind in their studies as a result. Both want to begin key essays and do sustained work on them so they can submit them on or before the deadline. John is committed to achieving this goal and is prepared to tolerate not attending a number of social events that he would like to attend in order to achieve it. In other words, he is willing to put up with the sacrifices that working towards achieving his goal would entail. Jack is also committed to achieving his goal but, unlike John, is not prepared to miss out on attending the same social events. In other words, Jack is not willing to put up with the sacrifices that pursuing his goal would entail. Who is more likely to achieve his goals, John or Jack? The answer is, of course, John.

Agreements about the REBT Focus

An idea that is widespread about therapy in general is that clients spend a lot of time talking about the past roots of their problems rather than their problems as they exist in the present. The idea here is that if clients understand how they acquired their problems in the first place, this will help them to address them in the present. However, REBT has attracted the opposing viewpoint: that when clients go to see REBT therapists, they talk about the present and the future but not about the past, and they focus on how they unwittingly maintain their problems rather than on how they originally acquired them. Help your clients to understand that while there is an element of truth about this latter view, it is not quite accurate. First of all, as an REBT therapist, you will encourage your clients to talk about whatever they are troubled about. So, if they are preoccupied with events in the past, then explain that you will help them to talk about such events. Having said that, you also need to explain that while REBT recognizes that your clients' past experiences contribute to their present problems, it also argues that their current rigid and extreme attitudes towards these experiences play a large role in why their problems persist.

Your clients, therefore, need to understand that while they will be allowed to discuss whatever they are preoccupied with in REBT, and while you will give due weight to the influence of the past on the present, a distinctive feature of REBT is that a clear focus will be placed on their current attitudes and how they currently behave as a way of helping them to address their problems effectively.

If you cannot agree on such a focus with some of your clients, then REBT may not be the right therapy for them. If so, discuss with them about making a judicious referral to a therapist who practises an approach that better meets such clients' ideas on the issue of what to focus on in therapy.

Agreements about the Therapist and Client Roles

I sometimes hear it said about therapy that it is a process that involves clients talking and therapists 'sorting out' the clients' problems. Some of your clients may also come to therapy with this expectation. This, of course, is very much at variance with what role you play as an REBT therapist and what role your clients are expected to play in REBT. The dominant view in

REBT is that the therapeutic relationship is a collaborative one, whereby you and your client work together in the service of your client's psychological health. However, both parties bring different resources to this collaboration, and in this section I will outline what these are. Collectively, these resources add up to your respective roles. It is important that you help your clients to understand these roles and agree to fulfil their role while you fulfil yours.

Your Role in REBT as a Therapist

Here is a list of what I consider your responsibilities are as an REBT therapist, which taken together constitute your role.

1. To bring your REBT knowledge to bear on the assessment and formulation of your client's problems and to communicate this clearly and explicitly.
2. To suggest and explain ways of tackling your client's problems, to make clear how these relate to the REBT-based assessment/formulation and how these ways will help your client to achieve their goals.
3. To engage your client as an active participant in a collaborative relationship where you work together in the service of your client's therapeutic goals.
4. To identify and respond to anything that your client is unclear about or has reservations about in the therapeutic process.
5. To identify potential and actual obstacles to client goal achievement and to deal with these in a sensitive way.
6. To set up what I call a meta-therapy dialogue, where you and your client stand back and discuss anything that pertains to the process of therapy; this is where you ask for client feedback about the therapeutic process and discuss your client's suggestions for modifications to their therapy with an open mind.

Your Clients' Role in REBT

Here is a list of what I consider to be your clients' responsibilities in REBT, which taken together constitute their role.

1. To speak openly about their problems, but to do so in a way and at a rate that is helpful for them.
2. To be active in the therapeutic process; to speak up and give their opinion about salient aspects of their therapy.

Your clients might think that, as you are the expert in REBT, you should know what you are doing and, thus, that if they don't understand a point you are making then that is their fault. Fortunately, this is a misguided view. It is misguided for a number of reasons which you may need to explain to your clients.

First, it assumes that you as REBT therapist can do no wrong. Explain that, since you are human first and a therapist a distant second, you are susceptible to all the vagaries of being human. In other words, you are fallible and can make mistakes and get things wrong. Even if you are a very skilled and experienced REBT therapist, you may, for example, explain something in a manner that your clients just don't understand.

Second, if you as therapist are infallible and always explain things in an understandable way, then it must be their fault if your clients don't understand a point that you make. The consequence of this view is that your clients are mainly in therapy to be the passive recipient of your wisdom as therapist and if they don't understand something, then there is no point in their bringing this to your attention, since the fault lies in them. Help your clients to see that again the reality is very different. REBT is a collaborative enterprise and you and your clients are equal participants in the therapeutic process. As you are both fallible, you both can get things wrong, and the best way that human beings have of putting things right is to communicate about them. Let's see what this means in practice.

Len, an REBT therapist, was seeing Julia about her performance anxiety. Len assessed Julia's problem and suggested a way of dealing with it, which Julia understood but did not fully agree with. Len intuited that Julia did not fully go along with his formulation and treatment suggestions, even though she claimed to do so.

Len: Julia, I sense that you may not fully agree with me that what I am calling 'over-preparing' your talk is a problem for you; am I right about this?

Julia: Well, I kind of see what you mean, but your suggestion that I limit my preparation to an hour a day is not something I am prepared to do. I'll limit it but not to an hour a day.

You can see from this brief vignette that Len is encouraging Julia to be a full participant in the therapy process, inviting her to speak up when she does not understand something or does not agree with something. In this way, Len is encouraging Julia to discharge her responsibility as a client.

While as an REBT therapist you value therapist–client collaboration, don't forget that you cannot check every point with your clients, so you need to rely to some extent on their speaking up and telling you when they don't understand something, don't agree with something or think that you have got things wrong. Help them to see that they have this responsibility and need to exercise it when necessary. Thus, if clients don't do this, it will increase the chances that 'obstacles to client change' will occur in therapy, which means that your clients will not make expected progress because in some way they silently have not signed on to certain key therapeutic points with which you thought they agreed. I will discuss this issue in the context of dealing with lack of progress in Chapter 7.

3. To undertake to carry out agreed tasks in the service of their goals (discussed in the next section and Chapter 6) and to be open about reasons why they did not do the tasks if this was the case.

If it transpires that there is not a good enough match between the therapist and client roles as outlined here and as preferred by both of you, then it is important to discuss this discrepancy with them and decide together what is the best way forward. If such an agreement about both of your roles cannot be made, then therapeutic progress will be severely compromised and you should help any such clients to seek help from a therapy that better approximates their views on such roles.

Agreements about Therapeutic Tasks

REBT involves you and your clients doing various things in therapy sessions and their doing things between therapy sessions to help them achieve their therapeutic goals. For the purposes of this discussion, I will refer to these as therapeutic tasks. Note well my point that both you and your clients are expected to carry out such tasks in REBT, and you should help your clients to understand this. What kind of agreements do you and your clients need to make about tasks in REBT, whether you do so explicitly or implicitly? Here are some of the main agreements that you and each client need to make with respect to therapeutic tasks.

- That you both understand what your respective tasks are and agree to implement them in the course of therapy.
- That you both understand how carrying out your respective tasks will help your client to achieve their therapeutic goals.

- That you both understand what your client's skills and capabilities are with respect to carrying out their therapeutic tasks and that you are both prepared to take the necessary steps to help them to implement these tasks if they cannot do so.
- That you both agree to make modifications to your respective tasks should it become necessary to do so.
- That you both understand that you will teach the client how to implement their tasks outside of therapy sessions and the more they do so, the more you will encourage them to take increasing responsibility to become their own therapist.

Agreements about Ending

I mentioned in the previous section that one of the issues that you and your clients need to agree on is when they will take increasing responsibility in therapy to become their own therapist. When this occurs, then you need to discuss with them how you are both going to end the process. There are a number of approaches to ending therapy in a planned way:

- Meet regularly (say weekly) and then set a date for the final session. A review session or sessions may or may not be scheduled.
- Decrease the frequency between sessions before setting a date for the final session. Again, a review session or sessions may or may not be scheduled.
- Decrease the frequency between sessions without setting a final date so that there are very long gaps between sessions, which effectively serve as review sessions.

Here as elsewhere, the important issue is that you agree with your clients on the best way to end the process for their own idiosyncratic situations.

In the next chapter, I discuss what you can do to help your clients to prepare themselves for therapy sessions so that they may derive the most benefit from them.

Chapter 4

Help Your Clients Prepare for Their REBT Sessions

Your clients may think that now that they are in therapy, all they need to do is turn up for their therapy sessions and talk. After all, isn't therapy supposed to be the talking cure? Well, yes and no! Obviously, your clients need to talk about what they are bothered about in their lives, but one way they can get the most out of therapy based on the principles of REBT is for them to come prepared for their therapy sessions. Your task is to help them to realize this and act on it.

What preparations you might help your clients make will, of course, depend on what problems they wish to discuss and the phase of therapy they are in. However, your clients might find the following guidelines helpful.

Encourage Clients to Develop Problem and Goal Lists

Developing a Problem List

Before clients attend their first therapy session, or as soon as possible after this session, you might suggest that they make a list of the problems they want to address in therapy. This is known as a 'problem list'. This means that when they contact you, in the first instance, to make an appointment, you might suggest that they develop such a list. When you are advising them to develop a problem list, encourage them to ensure that the problems on this list are those that *they* think they have and

DOI: 10.4324/9781003493150-5

that *they* want to address rather than problems that others think they have and want them to address in therapy. At this point, I suggest that you encourage clients to phrase these problems in their own words. If necessary, you can help them reword their problems so that they are expressed in a form that will best help them to tackle these problems. This normally involves you and your clients working to phrase their problems as clearly and specifically as possible.

As mentioned in the previous chapter, REBT works best if clients address problems that are within their direct control to change.

Developing a Goal List

You can also suggest that your clients develop a companion list of what *they* want to achieve from therapy with respect to these problems. So, for every problem they have listed, suggest that they set a goal. As they set their goals, help them to bear in mind that the presence of a healthy state is easier to achieve than the reduction or absence of a negative state. Thus, the goal 'I want to feel concerned about the possibility of being rejected' is easier for clients to achieve than 'I don't want to feel anxious about the possibility of being rejected'.

Again, suggest to your clients that they put their goals into their own words and tell them that you will, if necessary, help them to express these goals in a form that will best facilitate their achievement. When discussing goals with clients, it is useful to help them to understand one important point about therapy goals: that is, that your clients will probably not achieve them fully. I usually quote Marilyn Grey on this issue, who once said: 'No one ever has it "all together". That's like trying to eat once and for all.'

The same point that I made concerning targeting problems that are within your clients' direct control to change also applies to the topic of goals. The more your clients' goals are within their power to achieve, the more likely it is that they will achieve them. Ensure that they grasp this important point.

Suggest That Clients Come with a Clear Idea of What They Want to Discuss in Each Therapy Session

Your clients have met you and had an opportunity to tell you why they are seeking help, and you have decided to work together. They could just turn up for subsequent therapy sessions without doing any preparation, but in my view, they would not get as much out of these sessions as they would do if they came with a clear idea of what they want to discuss. Such client preparation can take a number of different forms, of which the following is a sample:

- Propose that they keep a log of events that they found upsetting in the week preceding their therapy session, perhaps suggesting that they put these events in some kind of order in which they want to discuss them.
- Suggest that they select a problem from their problem list that they want to address (known as the 'nominated problem') and encourage them to choose a specific example of that problem to discuss with you.
- Propose that they take a specific example of their nominated problem or a specific event about which they were upset and try to make sense of it using REBT's *ABC* framework.
- Encourage them to bring to the session anything that they want to revisit or did not understand from the previous session(s). This is an important point that I will address more fully in due course.

Session Agenda

You may wish to suggest that your clients develop an agenda for each therapy session that they attend. The purpose of this agenda is for you both to ensure that you cover what you want to deal with in the session and for you both to use session time effectively. In addition to the items mentioned in the previous section, agenda items for which they can prepare for before-hand include:

- One or more inventories that provide you both with an objective guide to how their mood is changing as a result of therapy (which may be completed just before the session, to save therapy time).
- A review of any between-session activities clients have agreed to do (discussed more fully in Chapter 6).

The important thing about the session agenda is that you and your clients use it flexibly, not rigidly. So, if something really important comes up in a session that is not on the agenda, your clients should have the freedom to explore it rather than have it ruled 'off limits' because it does not feature on the agenda.

Matters Arising

While I am not suggesting that an REBT session should be likened to a business meeting, if an agenda is to be set for therapy sessions, then it makes sense to have an item on that agenda entitled 'matters arising'. This means that you should encourage your clients to bring to the session anything that emerged from the previous session or the intervening period that they wish to discuss. This might include:

- Anything clients did not understand from the previous session.
- Anything clients disagreed with from the previous session.
- Any doubts, reservations or objections (DROs) clients had about the previous session or about therapy in general.

I will discuss this issue more fully in Chapter 7. In the next chapter, however, I will outline a process view of REBT that you can use with clients so that they can see how their therapy is likely to unfold.

Chapter 5

Help Your Clients Understand the Process of Change

Clients may find it helpful to have some idea of the process of change in REBT so that they can anticipate the process that lies ahead. As such, I am going to outline a number of stages that your clients may go through as they make progress on the problems for which they have sought REBT. You might share this framework with clients at the outset or as you both proceed, but whichever approach you take, it is important for clients to understand that these are not stages that they *must* go through or that the order in which I present them is the only or correct order. Rather, your clients should regard them as stages that they *may* go through, albeit perhaps in a different order to the one presented below.

Stage 1: Your Client Admits That They Have a Problem (or Problems) and They Accept Themselves for Having It (or Them)

While most people who seek REBT do so because they recognize that they have a problem, this is not universally the case. Thus, clients may have been sent for help or are consulting you because they consider that they have to, for some reason, rather than they want to do so. Indeed, clients may feel ambivalent about seeking help: part of them wants to, while another part of them does not. It is important that you encourage them to be honest with you about where they are on this issue so that they

DOI: 10.4324/9781003493150-6

can help themselves and you discover whether or not they have a problem, and if so, what might be stopping them from admitting to having it.

One of the major blocks to clients admitting that they have a problem is a sense of shame. Here, they believe something like: 'If I admit that I have this problem, then it would mean that I am weak, inadequate and worthless.' If this applies to a client, then help them to address this self-devaluation attitude idea before moving on to helping them to deal with the problem about which they feel ashamed.

Your clients may also devalue themselves even though they are readily able to admit to having a problem (which I refer to here as a 'primary problem'). While this 'meta-problem' (i.e. a problem about a problem) needs addressing at some point, once it has been disclosed to you, you should at this point help the client concerned to determine whether it needs therapeutic attention before you both address their primary problem or after you have done so. Basically, the more your clients' meta-problems interfere with their focusing their attention on their primary problems, either in therapy sessions or between them, the more likely it is that you and your clients need to address their meta-problems before their primary problems. I suggest that you outline such criteria to your clients so that they can understand your clinical thinking. However, here, as elsewhere in the therapy process, such decisions are made jointly between you and your client rather than unilaterally by you as therapist.

Stage 2: Your Client Understands Their Problems: Assessment and Formulation

Some REBT therapists prefer to have an idea of all the problems for which a client is seeking help and to understand the connections between them before helping the client to tackle these problems one at a time. This case formulation helps you to plan therapy based on an overall understanding of your client's problems and the mechanisms that are at play in their inter-connections. Of course, you will not carry out such a formu-lation without your client's active participation, and perhaps the most important thing about a case formulation is that it is arrived at jointly between you and your client. I regard this as a formulation-based approach to REBT.

Other REBT therapists will prefer to begin therapy by focusing on the problem the client wants to start with and will wait to discover the connections among their problems later. I regard this as a problem-based approach to REBT. In this approach, you will help your client and yourself to understand the dynamics of the problem that you both have selected to tackle first. This is known as problem assessment and, as with case formulation, you will encourage your clients to take an active role in this process by providing relevant information and agreeing on the assessment which you arrive at jointly.

Problem assessment and case formulation are carried out in both approaches, but the order in which they are done so is different. It is recommended that you explain to your cli-ents which approach you take so that they can understand what you are trying to do and thus actively participate in the process.

In my experience, most REBT therapists adopt a problem-based approach rather than a formulation-based approach to REBT. This stems from the view of the founder of REBT, Albert Ellis, who considered that it is best for REBT therapists to help clients with their problems straightaway, which, he argued, most clients seem to want.

From a working alliance perspective, if you, as an REBT therapist, do not have a preference concerning which approach to take with your clients, make each explicit to your clients and invite them to select the approach that they think will be most helpful to them.

Also, from a working alliance perspective, if you do have a preference concerning which approach to begin with, it is still important that you make this clear to your clients and get their agreement.

Stage 3: Your Client Focuses on One Problem at a Time and the Importance of Being Specific

Whether you adopt a formulation-based approach or a problem-based approach to REBT, when a client is ready to tackle their problems, suggest that they do so one at a time and, as they do so, encourage them to identify a specific example of the nominated problem. Explain to the client that the reason for this specificity is that, in general, it provides you both with more valuable information than if your client discusses their problems in general terms. You should invite your client to select a typical example of their nominated problem, a recent example, a vivid example or one that may occur in the near future. The important thing about the selected example is that it helps you both understand the factors that are at play in your client's nominated problem. In discussing this specific example of their nominated problem, help your client to do some or all of the following:

- Describe the situation in which the problem occurred and what they found most difficult about the situation.
- Identify what emotion(s) they felt in the situation.
- Identify how they acted in the situation or how they felt like acting.
- Identify what they did to try to cope with the problem.
- Set goals with respect to the problem. This will help them to know what they are aiming for in similar problematic situations.

Stage 4: Your Client Examines Rigid/ Extreme Attitudes and Develops Flexible/Non-Extreme Alternatives to These Attitudes and Associated Behaviour and Thinking

In REBT, rigid and extreme attitudes are seen to be at the core of people's emotional problems. These attitudes need to be need to be identified and examined, and flexible and non-extreme attitude alternatives need to be developed and adopted if change is going occur. It is vital that you help your clients to understand the role that such rigid and extreme attitudes have on their problems and that you both agree with how to deal with them.

It is important periodically to remind clients that in REBT, in addition to their rigid and extreme attitudes, they will be encouraged to consider the role that their behaviour and associated thinking play in their problems and will be helped to develop more constructive ways of acting and more realistic ways of thinking, as appropriate. It is my view that when clients' attitudes are flexible and non-extreme, their behaviour is constructive, their associated thinking is realistic and they marry the three consistently in dealing with what for them are adversities, then this constitutes the power of REBT.

Stage 5: Your Client Applies Their Learning

What clients learn within therapy sessions about the factors that account for the presence of their problems and how they unwittingly maintain them is, of course, a central plank of REBT, for without this they would continue to experience these problems, particularly if they are long-standing. However, unless clients apply what they learn from these sessions to their everyday lives, then it is unlikely that they will derive any lasting benefit from REBT. This is such an important topic that I have devoted an entire chapter to it (see Chapter 6).

Stage 6: Your Client Generalizes Their Gains to Other Problems

Once clients have made progress in dealing with their nominated problems, help them to generalize what they have learned to other problems that they would like help with.

Thus, imagine that one of your clients learned in therapy that their anxiety about meeting new people was based on their rigid and extreme attitude (e.g. 'I must not be rejected and if I am, that would be awful'). To deal with their anxiety, they avoided meeting new people. You can help this client to develop a flexible and non-extreme towards rejection (e.g., 'I don't want to be rejected, but it doesn't have to be the way I want. If I am rejected, that would be bad, but definitely not awful') and then to approach new people while practising this flexible/non-extreme attitude. If this is done effectively, your client should be able to meet new people and experience a significant decrease in their anxiety. If so, you can help them to apply their learning to their other anxieties, e.g. anxiety about public speaking and taking examinations. You can also encourage them to see that flexible and non-awfulizing thinking would also help with their jealousy problem, although they may have to learn some new skills in dealing with this latter problem as well.

Stage 7: Your Client Maintains Their Gains

It is tempting to think that once your clients have made significant progress in dealing with their problems, then therapy is over. However, given the fact that we humans seem to have a talent for lapsing (defined as making slips and returning briefly to the problem) and relapsing (defined as going back to square one), if clients do not deal adequately with these slips, then it is likely that they will relapse (see Chapter 8 for more information on this point). It is important, therefore, for you to help your clients recognize that they need to make a commitment to work consistently to maintain the benefits that they have made in therapy. Also, help them to appreciate that the more they practise what they have learned in therapy in a deliberate fashion, the more likely it is that these learnings will eventually become second nature to them.

Stage 8: Your Client Becomes Their Own REBT Therapist

There is an old adage which states: 'Give a person a fish and you feed them for a day. Teach a person to fish and you feed that person for a lifetime.' If we adapt this to REBT, we have: 'If you help your clients to solve a problem with REBT, then you will have helped them with that problem. If you teach them how to become their own REBT therapist, then you will have equipped them for life.' Thus, if it is feasible and they are interested, then the final stage of the REBT process involves you helping your clients to be their own REBT therapists. I will discuss this issue in Chapter 8.

At all stages of the change process, it is important that you appreciate and help your clients to appreciate that they will experience obstacles to change, and these need to be identified and addressed if you are going to help your clients to get the most out of REBT. I will deal with the most common obstacles to change in Chapter 7. Meanwhile, in the next chapter I will deal with a most important topic: how you can help your clients to get the most out of REBT in their everyday lives by encouraging them to apply there what they learn in therapy sessions.

Chapter 6

Help Your Clients Apply What They Learn

One of the most robust findings in the scientific literature on REBT and CBT is that clients who put into practice between sessions what they learn within sessions get more out of REBT than clients who don't do this between-session practice. It follows from this that if you want to help a client get the most out of REBT, then you need to encourage them to apply what they learn from therapy in their everyday life.

It is very important, in my view, that you help your clients realize fully that much of what they can achieve from REBT is within their hands and that making a commitment to undertake regular practice of whatever skills they have learned in their therapy sessions is crucial if they are going to derive the greatest benefit from REBT.

In dealing with this topic with my own clients, I give an example of such a commitment from my own life because I think that it details a number of points that are relevant to the importance of clients undertaking a similar commitment in REBT. You have my permission to use this with your own clients, or better still, use an example from your own life, as it will convey to your clients that you know from experience what you are talking about on this issue.

DOI: 10.4324/9781003493150-7

A number of years ago I was diagnosed with a disintegrating disc in my back and later with a torn cartilage in my right knee. I was told that while these two conditions might be helped with surgery, I could manage both myself by doing a number of relevant strengthening exercises. Practising these exercises takes me about 25 minutes every day. I decided from the outset that I would make a commitment to do such practice six days a week. I do so in the morning before I go for my jog-walk. My decision was underpinned by the following principles:

- I did not want to subject myself to surgery with its attendant risks and uncertain outcome.
- I wanted to take responsibility for my own recovery rather than handing over such responsibility to other people.
- I determined that I would do these exercises whether I wanted to do them or not. I realized that I didn't have to be or feel motivated to do the exercises. I just needed to do them. My behaviour was based on the following flexible/ non-extreme attitude: 'It would be nice if I feel motivated to do these exercises but I don't need such motivation. I can and will do them even if I don't feel motivated.'
- I learned to discriminate between good reasons for not doing the exercises (e.g. 'I am not going to do the exercises because I am ill') and rationalizations for not doing them (e.g. 'I will do the exercises tonight when I have more time to concentrate on them') and I resolved to respond to the latter and then take constructive action (i.e. by doing the exercises).
- I created favourable environmental conditions that would help me to do the exercises rather than hinder me from doing them. Thus, I set my alarm to help me to get up on time. I make sure that the room where I do the exercises is suitably heated and that the relevant equipment is to hand.

The five principles that I outlined above are very relevant to the issue of clients applying what they learn in REBT sessions to their everyday lives outside these sessions. Thus:

- The more your clients keep in mind the purpose of applying what they learn, the more they will do so. For example, suggest that they keep a clearly written reminder of their goals to hand to help them see the purpose of putting into practice what they have learned in therapy.
- The more your clients take responsibility for putting into practice what they learn in therapy, the more they tend to do this practice.
- If your clients resolve to put into practice what they learn in therapy, whether preferable conditions exist (e.g. having a feeling that they want to apply what they learn and having a sense of motivation for doing so) or not, then they are much more likely to do such practice than if they insist on the presence of such conditions.
- The more your clients monitor their thoughts relating to the possibility of their not putting what they have learned in REBT sessions into practice in their everyday lives and the more they learn to stand back and examine such thoughts, the more they will be able to discriminate between proper reasons for not taking action and rationalizations for not doing so. Once they become adept at making such discriminations, they will be able to respond productively to their rationalizations and thus they will probably choose not to act on their content.
- The more your clients structure their environment to help them take productive action, the more they will be able to do so. Structuring their environment depends, in part, on their understanding how to get the best out of themselves with respect to putting their REBT-derived learning into practice.

  Thus, I am more likely to write when I am in an environment where there is non-intrusive noise and hustle and bustle around me (e.g. while the TV is on or in a coffee bar) than when I am in a silent environment. Consequently, I write while the TV is on or I seek out coffee bars in which to write. Help your clients to think about the importance of structuring their environment when planning to put into practice what they have learned from your REBT sessions and help them to choose an environment, if possible, that will help them maximize the chances that they will do this practice.

Homework Tasks

You may refer to activities that clients undertake to put into practice what they have learned in therapy sessions as 'homework tasks'. Be aware, though, that some clients do not like the term 'homework' given the negative connotations that it has for them with respect to their school experiences, for example. If this is the case for some of your clients, select together a term that is more acceptable to them.

In this section, I will deal with two main issues: (i) negotiating homework tasks with clients and (ii) reviewing homework tasks with them.

Negotiating Homework Tasks with Your Clients

With respect to negotiating homework tasks with your clients, you can help them get the most out of these tasks if you do the following:

Negotiate homework tasks with your clients. Refrain from unilaterally telling a client what to do for homework between therapy sessions. Rather, negotiate a suitable homework task with them.

Help ensure that each homework task is a relevant one. Such a task should follow logically from what you and your client have discussed in the therapy session. It may involve your client reading something, identifying attitudes, examining such attitudes, imagining acting differently or actually doing so. The type of homework task negotiated should also be relevant to the stage reached by the two of you on the problem or issue you are working on together.

Ensure that your clients understand the nature of negotiated tasks and their therapeutic purpose. Check that your clients understand what they have agreed to for homework and the purpose of so doing. Ask them to put this into their own words. If your clients don't understand what they have agreed to do or why they have agreed to do it, they are unlikely to get much out of the task even if they do it.

Work with your clients to select homework tasks that are 'challenging, but not overwhelming' for them. Help your client choose a task that is not too easy for them (and thus of very limited therapeutic power) or too difficult for them (in which case they are unlikely to do it). A task that is challenging but not overwhelming for them avoids these two unhelpful extremes and maximizes the benefits your client is likely to derive from the selected task.

Introduce and explain the 'no lose' concept of homework tasks to your clients. It is useful to explain to your client that if they do the negotiated homework task, then that is good because it is likely that they have benefitted from doing so, and if they don't do the task, good can come out of that too, since this will help you both to understand more about the nature of their problem and the obstacle(s) to making progress. I will discuss this latter issue in Chapter 7.

Ensure that your clients have the necessary skills to carry out the homework tasks and believe that they can do them. If a client lacks the skills to carry out a homework task, then no amount of determination will make up for this lack. If your client does lack certain skills that are important for them to acquire before they do the task, then you should determine that this is the case and help them to acquire the requisite skills. If, on the other hand, you think that they have such skills in their repertoire but don't have the confidence to use them, then you should address this issue, helping them to see that they don't need such confidence in order to put their skills into practice. Here, it is useful to help clients to understand that confidence often comes from doing things unconfidently and learning from the resultant experiences.

Allow sufficient time in sessions to negotiate homework tasks properly with your clients. Novice REBT therapists know that they 'should' negotiate homework tasks with their clients but often lose track of time in therapy and realize, often very late, that the therapy session is ending and they have not helped their clients set homework. Consequently, they panic and often end up by unilaterally 'giving' their clients homework tasks rather than taking their time to negotiate such tasks properly with their clients. To safeguard against this happening, be mindful of the passage of time and manage sessions sufficiently to enable you to spend time negotiating suitable homework tasks with your clients.

Elicit firm commitments from your clients that they will carry out homework tasks. It is one thing for a client to agree to carry out a homework task; it is another thing for them to commit themself to doing so. Thus, ask them to make a firm commitment to do the task that you have both negotiated and to explore any reluctance that they have to do so.

Help your clients specify when, where and how often they will carry out homework tasks. The more specific you can help your client to be concerning when, where and how often they will carry out the negotiated homework task, the more likely it is that they will do so. Thus, ask your clients to give such specific undertakings. Otherwise, they may be tempted to delay carrying out the task, perhaps leaving it till the last minute. If this happens, it will mean, in all probability, that they won't get the most out of doing the agreed task.

Encourage your clients to make written notes of homework tasks and their relevant details and to refer to them when appropriate. When clients do not carry out their homework tasks, one of the main reasons they give is that they forgot what the homework was and that they hadn't made a written note of the task. Thus, ask your client to make a written note of the agreed task and suggest that they refer to this written note periodically so that they do not forget what it was when they come to do it.

Elicit from your clients the potential obstacles to homework completion and help them deal in advance with any such obstacles. In the next chapter, I will discuss the more general issue of why clients may not be making as much progress in REBT as you and they may reasonably expect. One of the main reasons for lack of progress is failure to complete homework tasks. Thus, explore with your clients, in advance, possible obstacles to homework task completion and how these might be dealt with. If they have continued difficulty in carrying out such tasks, I suggest that you ask them to fill out the form in Appendix 3 and discuss their responses with them.

Help your clients to rehearse homework tasks in their sessions, if practicable. If doing so is practicable, and there is sufficient time, then suggest that your client rehearse their agreed homework task in the therapy session. The reason for this is twofold. First, it gives them the experience of doing the task in controlled conditions so they can get a sense of what doing it in the outside world might be like. Second, it may help you both to identify and problem-solve an obstacle to carrying out the task not already identified.

Reviewing Homework Tasks with Your Clients

Unless you review homework tasks with your clients in subsequent sessions, it is unlikely that your clients will consider them to have the level of importance that they actually have in REBT. Again, it is worthwhile keeping in mind that one of the most robust research findings in REBT and CBT is that clients who routinely carry out homework tasks get a lot more out of the process than those who do not. With this in mind, with respect to reviewing homework tasks with a client, I suggest that you do the following:

Check with your client whether or not they did the home-work task. Unless you check with your client concerning whether or not they did the task and what their experiences of doing so were, then you will be implicitly communicating to them that doing such tasks are not important in REBT when, in reality, they are. Initiate such a review at the beginning of the next session and explain to the client that you will do this. Encourage them, therefore, to prepare in advance of the session what to say about doing (or not doing) the task, as I discussed in Chapter 4.

Determine the reason(s) why your client did not do the task as agreed, if this was the case, and address with them any obstacles. If your client did not do the homework task, then explore with them the reasons for this. You might encourage them to prepare for this discussion by suggesting that they complete the form to be found in Appendix 3 and bring their responses to therapy. Your best stance here should be to be genuinely interested in identifying any obstacles to home-work completion with a view to helping your clients to address these obstacles rather than to reprimand them for not doing the task.

Check whether your client made any modification(s) to the task and, if so, determine the reasons for the modification(s). Your client may have done their homework task and they may have thought they had done so successfully, but they may have changed the task to make it easier for them to carry it out. In doing so, they may have reduced the thera-peutic power of the task. Given this, enquire in some detail about what your client actually did to determine whether or not this was the case. If it was, help them to discover what led them to make the modification and deal with this factor if it helps them unwittingly to maintain their problem. It is important that you both acknowledge what your client achieved by doing the task as well as pointing out to them the problems raised by the modification they made to it.

Bernice agreed to deal with her anxiety about going shopping and losing control in supermarkets by practising her newly developed flexible/non-extreme attitude towards not feeling in control and doing so on her own in a supermarket without access to support from others. She reported that she did this and that the prospect of losing control seemed more manageable. However, on closer questioning, Bernice admitted that during the task she had phoned her daughter for support and even though she did not speak to her daughter, she gained support from knowing that her daughter was there on the open phone line should she need her. How would you respond to Bernice here if you were her therapist?

What her therapist did was to acknowledge the stride forward that Bernice had made by going to the supermarket on her own, but discussed with her that she only thought that she could do so if she had direct contact with her daughter. This led to an exploration of Bernice's thoughts about doing the task without such support and they negotiated a new task where she went to the supermarket without her mobile phone based on the work she and her therapist did on the thoughts she had about the original task.

Review what your client learned from doing the task. Your client doing the task as agreed is important, of course, but what they learned from doing so is, in some ways, more important. So, ask your client what they learned from doing the task. Sometimes what they learned may not be that helpful to them. Thus, a client may learn from giving a public speech as a homework task that nobody laughed at them and that nobody will laugh when they give a talk. While it may be good for the client to learn that nobody laughed when they predicted that everybody would, it is unreasonable for them to jump to the conclusion that nobody will laugh in future. Here, you might suggest to the client that it would be helpful to prepare to be laughed at even though this event may be unlikely.

Help your client deal with homework 'failure'. Your client may have done the task and derived no benefit from it and thus may consider the homework to have been a failure. As discussed earlier in this section, there are times when you will carefully examine what your client did, what happened and their thinking about the experience, and exploring homework 'failure' is one of those times. Remember what I said earlier in this chapter about the 'no lose' concept of homework completion. If one of your client's homework tasks was a 'failure', then that is bad, but the good thing to come out of it is understanding why it failed and using what you and your client discovered in this process to help the latter more effectively in the future.

Capitalize on your client's successes. While I have concentrated on some of the difficulties that your clients might experience in the area of homework tasks in REBT, I want to stress that very often clients do their tasks as agreed and gain a lot from doing so. When this happens, help them to capitalize on their successes and to use their derived learning to further their progress on the problems that they are focusing on and perhaps to employ this learning with other problems as well.

Your clients applying what they learn from therapy sessions to their everyday lives is the heart of REBT, in my view. However, as we have seen, REBT does not always go smoothly, and in the next chapter, I will focus on the issues that emerge when your clients don't make the expected progress from therapy.

Chapter 7

Help Your Clients Understand and Deal with Lack of Progress

Sometimes in therapy, clients do not make the progress that they can be expected to have made. If this occurs, invite your client to join you in looking for reasons for such lack of progress and in dealing with these obstacles to change accordingly. In this chapter, I will consider some of the common reasons for lack of progress and suggest ways in which you can best deal with them.[1] I will use the following structure in this chapter:

- Lack of client progress due to problems in the working alliance.
- Lack of client progress due to client factors.
- Lack of client progress due to therapist factors.

I will discuss the most common obstacles to progress that occur in each of the above categories before discussing the more general issue of how you and your clients can address such obstacles.

Lack of Client Progress due to Problems in the Working Alliance

A good working alliance between you and your clients is what sustains therapy over the course, and thus if one of your clients is not making expected progress, it is important that you and your client investigate the possibility that there is a problem in the alliance that needs addressing.

DOI: 10.4324/9781003493150-8

The Therapeutic Bond Between You and Your Client Is Not Good

The bonding aspect of the working alliance concerns the feeling tone that exists in the relationship between you and your client. Thus, if you don't have good feelings for one another, this may have a negative effect on your client's progress. My view is that while your client can still make progress in therapy if you and your client don't like one another, it is more difficult to do so if there is no mutual respect or if your client does not have confidence in your expertise. If either of these situations occurs then you need to address the issues explicitly in order to resolve them. If they can't be resolved, you will need to refer the client to a different therapist

The Therapeutic Bond Between You and Your Client Is Too Good

You may think it strange that getting on too well might be a reason why your client may not be making expected progress in REBT, but it certainly can happen. You and your client may enjoy each other's company so much that you may drift away from the primary objective concerning why they are seeking therapy – to address your client's emotional problems. If this happens then you need to refocus the therapy towards emotional problem-solving and away from having pleasant interchanges that may not help the client solve their problems.

I introduced the following points in Chapter 3 when I was talking about the therapeutic agreements that you need to make with your clients in REBT, but since disagreements on these points may explain lack of expected client progress, I will discuss them briefly here (see also Chapter 3). Please note that while the disagreements that I discuss below may be clear and explicitly stated, they are more often implicit and therefore not stated.

You and Your Client Disagree on the Nature of the Problem(s)

If your client considers that they have a problem with guilt, for example, while you consider that their problem is one of shame, you may end up talking at cross purposes, and since these two emotions are underpinned by different attitudes and associated with different behaviours and thinking, this may result in you focusing on the wrong factors and therefore in lack of progress. In this case, you need to discuss the client's nominated problem and develop a shared understanding before working to find a solution to the problem.

You and Your Client Disagree about the Goals of Therapy

You and your client may agree on the nature of their problem, but may disagree concerning the goals of therapy with respect to this problem. Thus, you both may agree that your client has a problem with unhealthy suppressed anger, for example, but while your client may think that the goal of therapy should be to help them get this anger out of their system, you may think that the goal should be to help your client to express themself with respectful annoyance. If this is the case, you will be going in one direction while your client will be going in another, which again may result in lack of progress. Address this with your client if this is the case and develop shared goals.

You and Your Client Have Disagreements about the Focus of Therapy

While nothing is ruled out when it comes to your client discussing their problems, as I pointed out in Chapter 1, the focus of REBT is largely on the present and the future, and when the past is discussed it is done so in a way that facilitates understanding of these two foci. Thus, if your client wants to discuss their past experiences extensively without regard to the present and the future, then they may not make progress if you do not join them in a comprehensive examination of their past. REBT theory would also hypothesize that your client may not make much progress even if you do join them in this exploration, since while you are going over the past with them, they are still being influenced by the attitude and behavioural factors that underpin their problems both in the present and going forward into the future. If this occurs, discuss this with your client and develop a shared focus.

You and Your Client Disagree about Your Respective Roles

As discussed in Chapter 3, REBT involves you and your client both adopting an active and collaborative role in therapy, and when this does not happen for any reason, your client may not make as much therapeutic progress as when it does. While the most common occurrence on this issue concerns your client not assuming an active role, it may happen that you may also not be active in the process or may fail to be sufficiently collaborative with the client. If this occurs, take steps to develop a more collaborative relationship and then encourage their more active engagement in the therapeutic process. If necessary, you may need to encourage yourself to get more actively involved in the process.

You and Your Client Disagree about Therapeutic Tasks or Experience Other Problems about These Tasks

Therapeutic tasks are activities that you and your client engage in with the purpose of helping the latter achieve their therapeutic goals. If you both do not agree that undertaking these tasks is helpful, then this may compromise your client's progress. Even if you do agree on this point, things may go wrong, as shown in the following vignette.

> Gerald was seeking help from an REBT therapist for depression and readily agreed with the REBT-based conceptualization of his problems. His therapist taught him to use a form that was designed to help people identify and respond to rigid and extreme attitudes that underpin depression, and Gerald could see the sense of doing this. However, Gerald had very poor spelling, about which he was ashamed, and this resulted in his not completing the forms as requested by his therapist. His sense of shame prevented him from bringing up this obstacle with his therapist.

Raise task-related issues with your client and encourage them to engage only in tasks that make sense to them.

Lack of Client Progress due to Client Factors

When I say that your client may be largely responsible for their own lack of progress, it is not to blame them but to help you address such obstacles with them fair and square. With that in mind, let's look at some common client obstacles to change. If this is the case, you need to help the client to identify reasons for their pessimistic view of change and address them with the client.

Your Client Believes That Change Is Not Possible

If your client thinks that change is not possible, they will not engage fully with the REBT process. Consequently they will not get as much out of the process as they would do if they thought that they could change.

Your Client Opts for Short-Term 'Solutions' to Their Problem(s)

We, as human beings, generally seek to make ourselves comfortable whenever we experience discomfort, and this is not a problem for us as long as there is no good reason for experiencing such discomfort. Since achieving therapeutic goals generally involves discomfort, then unless your client is prepared to experience such discomfort their progress will be very limited. Signs that your client is opting for the short-term solution of getting rid of the discomfort associated with their problem rather than being prepared to experience discomfort in the short term while facing their problem and dealing with it are many, but include: denying that they have a problem, overcompensating for their problem and using safety-seeking behaviours to avoid experiencing their problem.

Luke was anxious about meeting new people, especially in social settings. In order to deal with this problem, Luke would (i) avoid such occasions, or if he could not do so, he would (ii) pretend that he had lost his voice so he did not have to speak to people. He would also (iii) consume quite a lot of alcohol to 'take the edge off' his anxiety, as he put it. In REBT, his therapist helped him to see that while these three behaviours kept his anxiety at bay in the short term, they did not help him deal with his anxiety problem in the longer term. Luke learned more adaptive ways of dealing with his anxiety by developing a set of flexible/non-extreme attitudes and resolved to put this learning into practice rather than use the three short-term 'solutions'. However, Luke did not make as much progress as possible because it transpired that he managed to get one of his friends invitations to these social events and spent time with that person rather than talking to people whom he did not know while practising the REBT skills that he learned in his therapy sessions and agreed to practise for homework.

With such clients, you need to encourage them both to keep their long-term objectives at the forefront of their minds and to bear the discomfort of working towards their goals.

Your Client Has Doubts, Reservations and Objections to Aspects of Their Therapy That They Do Not Disclose

REBT is based on a particular way of making sense of your client's problems, of explaining how they may have unwittingly maintained these problems and of determining what they need to do to address them effectively. In order to get the most out of REBT, your client needs to collaborate with you in developing these problem-based and therapy-based understandings. When your client doesn't make as much progress as expected, it may be due to one or more DROs that they have with respect to these understandings that they have not expressed, the existence of which has negatively affected their participation in therapy. For this reason, I urge you to be vigilant for the existence of such DROs and to enquire about their existence at regular intervals.

Carol had a problem with chronic guilt and was easily manipulated by others, with the result that she would always put others before herself. She worked closely with her REBT therapist to develop an REBT-based conceptualization of her problems, and together, they worked to devise a way of addressing these problems effectively. However, despite doing all her agreed homework tasks, Carol did not make much progress in therapy. After therapy finished, Carol admitted to her friend that she had several doubts about the treatment plan that she, at least on the surface, was involved in developing with her therapist. She told her friend that she did not tell her therapist her doubts because she did not want to upset her therapist. This was the case even though her therapist had asked her if she had any doubts, reservations or objections to any aspect of therapy.

Your Client Thinks That Intellectual Insight Is Enough to Help Them

In REBT there are two forms of insight, what might be termed 'intellectual insight' and 'emotional insight'. When your client has intellectual insight, they understand and agree with the REBT concepts that they are being taught but this insight has not yet impacted their feelings and behaviour. Emotional insight, on the other hand, does impact on your client's feelings and behaviour. Thus, they know that making an important error does not make them a less worthwhile person, but this insight (intellectual) will not impact on their feelings and behaviour until they act on it and do so until they come to believe it. Thus, your client may not make much progress in REBT if they believe that intellectual insight is enough. If so, you need to address this misconception until they can see that only emotional insight will help them achieve their goals and maintain their progress.

Your Client Is Not Prepared to Work for Change

As I have discussed throughout this book, REBT depends on your client taking an active role in the therapeutic process both inside and outside the therapy room. So, if they are not prepared to work for change, then they will not make very much progress. Here are some common progress-blocking attitudes that clients have in this area:

- 'I shouldn't have to help myself; it is my therapist's job to help me.'
- 'I'm too lazy to help myself.'
- 'I don't have the time to carry out homework tasks.'

If your client holds these or similar attitudes, you need to discuss them with the person and encourage them to re-engage in therapy as a more active participant.

Your Client Is Intolerant of the Discomfort and Unfamiliarity Associated with Change

While your client can achieve a lot from REBT, they will not do so (i) unless they are prepared for the discomfort of facing up to and discussing painful issues and (ii) unless they are prepared to tolerate the unfamiliarity that they will experience during the process of change. As I often say to my clients: 'If it isn't strange, it isn't change.' So, if your client is intolerant of such discomfort and feelings of unnaturalness, then they will not make much progress in REBT, and to remedy this, you need to discuss this with your client and encourage them to bear the 'strange' feelings until they fade.

Lack of Client Progress due to Therapist Factors

So far, I have discussed possible reasons why your client has not made expected progress in REBT that are due to problems in the working alliance that you have with your client or to factors within the client themself. However, you may be largely responsible for your client's lack of progress, and I will briefly discuss some of these therapist factors in this section.

The Therapist Lacks Important General Therapeutic Skills

One of the most common therapist factors that impedes client progress is that the therapist lacks general therapeutic skills. When a therapist lacks general therapeutic skills:

- They fail to listen to their client or empathize with them.
- They consistently put words into their client's mouth.
- They interact with their client in a way that reinforces the client's problems (e.g. they are too active, and this reinforces their client's problematic passivity).

- They have unreasonably high or unreasonably low expectations of their client, which results in them either pushing the client too much or too little.
- They are too forceful in making points and fail to elicit or take into account their client's views.
- They misjudge what stage of change their client is in and work with them in the wrong stage of change (e.g. they assume that the client is ready to change something when they are, in fact, ambivalent about doing so).

The Therapist Lacks REBT-Specific Skills

One of the other most common therapist factors that impedes client progress is that the therapist lacks REBT-specific skills. When a therapist lacks such skills:

- They fail to understand accurately their client's problems in REBT terms.
- They fail to explain clearly their understanding of their client's problems even if this may be accurate.
- They fail to suggest an REBT approach that, if they and the client both use properly, will help the client deal effectively with their problems.
- They suggest an effective REBT approach to the client's problems but implement this poorly.
- They are poor in negotiating and reviewing suitable homework tasks.
- They do not identify and address effectively reasons why the client may not be making expected progress in REBT.

The Therapist Has Personal Issues/Problems Which Interfere with Them Helping Their Client

Therapists are human and are not immune from the problems and issues that all human beings are capable of experiencing.

Having said that, hopefully, whatever problems an REBT therapist may have will not intrude on the client's therapy. Sadly, this is not always the case, and here are some examples where the therapist's issues/problems do interfere with therapy and may help to explain the client's lack of progress:

- The therapist has the same problem as their client and has not been able to help themself with that problem, with the result that they fail to offer their client credible help.
- The therapist believes that they need their client's approval, with the result that they fail to confront the client appropriately.
- The therapist believes that their worth depends on their client's progress, with the result that they may get angry or defensive if the client does not make the progress that the therapist expects.
- They have a problem with impatience and seem to get impatient or irritable if their client fails to understand something or when therapy does not go smoothly.
- They disturb themself about their client's problems, with the result that they cannot gain the professional distance they need to help the client effectively.

As I will discuss below, all these therapist factors need to be addressed in supervision or personal therapy. If any apply to you, please take the appropriate remedial action.

Dealing with Lack of Progress

When your clients are not making as much progress as they might reasonably expect for one or more of the reasons discussed above (or for other reasons), it is important that you and your client address this issue. If you do not do so, it is unlikely that your clients will be able, on their own, to overcome these obstacles to progress.

Most people would say, rightly, in my view, that it is mainly your responsibility as a therapist to initiate a discussion concerning these reasons, even if your client has brought up the issue of lack of progress in the first place. However, your client also has a responsibility to speak up, since you as therapist will not be able to read their mind and deal with matters without their active participation in this process. I will discuss both your and your client's responsibility for dealing with lack of progress in the rest of this chapter.

Your Responsibility for Dealing with Lack of Client Progress

If you think that your client is not making progress as expected, then it is important that you bring this to their attention and initiate a discussion about this. You should preferably also initiate such a discussion when your client has brought up the issue of lack of progress. When you initiate such a discussion, then this will go better if you have already established what is known as a 'meta-therapy dialogue' with your client, as discussed earlier in the book (see Chapter 3). This refers to a process where you and your client stand back, as it were, and reflect on issues pertaining to therapy. If you have already set up such a dialogue with your client, then the subsequent discussion about lack of progress should go more smoothly than if such a dialogue has not yet been established.

Once the discussion about lack of progress has been initiated, there are two major things that you need to do to increase the chances that this discussion will be fruitful.

You Need to Adopt a Flexible and Negotiable Stance in the Discussion

When you do adopt such a flexible stance, then your client will say things like:

- 'My therapist and I are good at finding a solution if we disagree.'

- 'I do not feel that I have to pretend to agree with my therapist's goals for our therapy so that the sessions run smoothly.'
- 'I feel like I have a say regarding what we do in therapy.'
- 'My therapist is flexible and takes my wants or needs into consideration.'
- 'I do not feel that my therapist tells me what to do and has regard for my wants or needs.'
- 'My therapist is flexible in their ideas regarding what we do in therapy.'

As you can see from the above statements when you establish a flexible and negotiable stance, this will help both of you to reflect on the reasons for your client's lack of expected progress. Compare this with what your client is likely to say if you are rigid and not open to negotiation about possible reasons for your client's lack of progress.

- 'I feel that my therapist tells me what to do, without much regard for my wants or needs.'
- 'My therapist is inflexible and does not take my wants or needs into consideration.'
- 'My therapist is rigid in their ideas regarding what we do in therapy.'
- 'I feel like I do not have a say regarding what we do in therapy.'
- 'I pretend to agree with my therapist's goals for our therapy so the session runs smoothly.'
- 'My therapist and I are not good at finding a solution if we disagree about what we should be working on in therapy.'

Indeed, if you routinely display such closed mindedness, this may be a prime reason for your client's lack of progress. Most therapists at times show a closed-minded attitude, but if you do so routinely, then you may need help from your supervisor, or if it is rooted in personal issues, you should consult your own therapist.

You Need to Demonstrate That You Are Comfortable
Dealing with Disagreement and with Any Negative Feelings
That Your Client Might Express

When you demonstrate such comfort, then your client will say
things like:

- 'I feel that I can disagree with my therapist without harming
  our relationship.'
- 'My therapist encourages me to express any concerns I have
  with our progress.'
- 'I am comfortable expressing disappointment in my therapist
  when it arises.'
- 'My therapist encourages me to express any anger I feel
  towards them.'
- 'My therapist is able to admit when they are wrong about
  something we disagree on.'
- 'I am comfortable expressing frustration with my therapist
  when it arises.'

As you can see from these statements, if you can comfortably
hear and, indeed, invite your client's negativity about aspects of
the therapy and the way in which you are working with them,
they are likely to feel able, in turn, to be honest about their
negative feelings about their lack of progress and the things that
may be hindering such progress. Your client will also feel free
to say what they don't like about the therapy.

Compare this with what your client is likely to say if you are
uncomfortable dealing with disagreement and with their negative feelings about you or therapy.

- 'I don't feel that I can disagree with my therapist without
  harming our relationship.'
- 'My therapist does not encourage me to express any concerns
  I have with our progress.'

- 'I am not comfortable expressing disappointment in my therapist when it arises.'
- 'My therapist does not encourage me to express any anger I feel towards them.'
- 'My therapist is unable to admit when they are wrong about something we disagree on.'
- 'I am not comfortable expressing frustration with my therapist when it arises.'

The chances are that in such circumstances, your client will be reluctant to be honest about their thoughts and feelings about why they may not be progressing in therapy. Most therapists at times show discomfort about disagreement and about hearing something negative about therapy, but again, if you do so routinely, you may need supervisory and/or therapeutic help.

You Need to Give Your Client Honest Feedback about How Therapy Is Proceeding and What Factors Might Explain Their Lack of Progress

As well as being able to take bad news as demonstrated above, you also need to be able to give bad news in offering your opinion about why your client may not be making expected progress. A good therapist has the ability to be honest without discouraging their clients in the process. Thus, if you consider that a major reason for your client's lack of progress is their failure to apply themself in a consistent way to carrying out homework tasks, then you should say so, but in a way that shows that your client could apply themself and, as importantly, in a way that engages them in an honest exploration of why they may not be applying themself as consistently as they might. I should add that it is particularly important for you to be honest if your client has unreasonable expectations about change and that they are, in fact, making as much progress as they might be expected to be making. Encouraging your client to develop more realistic expectations about progress may help them to re-invest in the process of REBT and make advances in a slower, but perhaps more sustained, manner.

If you do not give your client genuine feedback, you may be depriving them of the opportunity to address some uncomfortable truths which, if addressed, may well help them to make more progress in therapy.

How You Might Discharge Your Responsibility for Lack of Client Progress due to Therapist Factors

I think that there are four forums in which you can explore obstacles to your clients' progress that stem from your own factors as a therapist.

1. Supervision
   Clinical supervision involves you regularly consulting a more experienced REBT therapist or one of equal experience, where you can raise and discuss the factors that emanate largely from you which serve as possible obstacles to client progress. Such factors relate largely to issues to do with clinical skills or personal issues which are focused on particular clients and are not general in nature. In using clinical supervision in this way, you need to be able to trust your supervisor to respect you even though you may disclose information about yourself which may conflict with your therapeutic ideals. Clinical supervision should help you to identify your blind spots as a practitioner and to go back to address obstacles to client progress with greater insight and in an enthusiastic manner.
2. Personal reflection
   You may also derive benefit from personally reflecting on the difficulties you encounter as an REBT therapist as they pertain to lack of client progress that can be attributed to you as a person and/or a therapist. While perhaps less disciplined and less structured than supervision, such personal reflection

is particularly suited to you if you can be honest with yourself and find such introspection creative in identifying and dealing with the personal factors that may account for the lack of client progress.

3. Peer consultation

While less professionally accountable and less formal than supervision, peer consultation – which involves you consulting a trusted colleague on an 'as needed' basis – may provide you with a safe space to discuss problems that you might experience as a therapist where you are largely responsible for your client's lack of expected progress. Such peer consultations tend to be two way, and at other times your peer may consult you on their own difficulties with clients. Where confrontation occurs, it is done within a context of mutual trust and professional respect.

4. Personal therapy

When you notice that you have recurring personal issues with some clients which result in their making less than expected progress, then personal therapy is the best forum for exploration and examination. If the therapist that you consult for your personal therapy has expertise in working with therapists experiencing similar difficulties, then so much the better.

Your Client's Responsibility for Dealing with Lack of Progress

Having outlined what responsibility you have in dealing with your client's lack of progress, let me be clear and state that your client also has responsibility here. This involves your client speaking up and being honest. While you as a therapist need to facilitate your client in this regard (a) by creating a climate which fosters such expressions of honesty and (b) by educating your client in seeing that such honesty is an integral part of the client role, your client still has a choice whether or not to speak up and be honest. They may well be apprehensive about being assertive in this regard for fear of hurting your feelings, for example, but if they do not take the risk, particularly when you have demonstrated your flexibility and comfort in dealing with difficult issues, then remember this: you can't help your client with something about which you do not know.

However, if your client doesn't feel able to speak up and be honest about something that may be hindering their progress in therapy, then you might encourage them to talk about their difficulty about doing so. You can help in two ways as a therapist. First, you can help your client overcome their fear of speaking up, and second, when they have spoken up, you can help them with whatever they have spoken up about.

Violet was seeking help for a chronic problem with procrastination. She was making good progress with this until her therapist put forward the hypothesis that a component of her problem was due to autonomy issues. She privately disagreed with this hypothesis but told her therapist that she agreed. It was when she stopped making progress that her therapist encouraged a discussion about possible reasons for this. During this discussion, Violet told her therapist that she found it difficult to be honest with him. He helped her to investigate this with him and this then encouraged her to tell him that she thought he was wrong about his autonomy hypothesis. He demonstrated comfort with this feedback, and with therapy properly recalibrated, she began to make progress again.

By identifying and addressing the reasons for your client's lack of progress, you should be able to help them get back on track, make progress and eventually achieve their goals. When this happens, it may be time to end therapy with your client. However, you also have the possibility, if practicable, of helping them to become their own REBT therapist, and I will discuss this issue in the following chapter.

Note

1   In this chapter, when I discuss lack of progress, I refer to instances when your clients are not making as much progress as they might reasonably be expected to be making. They may, of course, have unreasonable expectations of progress with respect to their problems and are, in fact, making expected progress – in which case, you will want to discuss this with your clients, as I will make clear later in the chapter.

Chapter 8

Help Your Clients Become Their Own REBT Therapist

One of the major goals that you are likely to have is to help your clients to become their own REBT therapist. This means that you will help them to develop a number of skills which you will encourage them to use increasingly for themselves over the course of therapy, with the aim of continuing to do so when formal therapy has ended.

While this is a major aim of REBT, it is important to note that your clients may or may not be interested in learning to use REBT-based self-help skills for themselves after therapy has ended, or, if they are, they may be interested in doing this informally in their own way and may not wish to learn these skills in a more structured, formal way. The important point, and one that I have stressed throughout this book, is that effective REBT therapists are prepared to tailor their approaches according to their clients' idiosyncratic situations and preferences. Having said that, in this final chapter, I am going to discuss what you can do to help clients who are interested in learning how to become their own REBT therapist. In doing so, I will not discuss specific skills that may or may not be relevant to your clients; rather, I will focus on categories of skills that are likely to have broader relevance.

DOI: 10.4324/9781003493150-9

Helping Your Clients to Learn Assessment Skills

When you help a client to work towards becoming their own REBT therapist, it is important that you help them learn how to identify the important factors that comprise their reactions to situations that are problematic for them. As part of this process, you may suggest that they use a printed form on which there will be a number of headings and spaces under those headings for them to write down their responses. There are a number of such forms, and the one you suggest may be dictated by your preferences as a therapist and/or the nature of your client's problem(s) for which they are seeking help.

Assessment forms are usually designed to help your client to assess specific information. They may or may not include information detailing how to complete them. Once a client has filled out such a form on a number of occasions, you will be able to discern and help them see more general patterns emerge that will help them to anticipate how they may respond so that they can help themself early on in a problem episode or even in advance of a likely episode. I will discuss this in greater detail later in this chapter.

When your clients are learning to assess their problems, you can help them to do the following:

- Identify the kind of situations they find difficult (e.g. speaking in public).
- Identify what they find particularly disturbing about these situations (e.g. their mind going blank). This is their adversity at A.
- Identify the main troublesome emotions at C that they experience in these situations and the major physiological expressions of these feelings, if relevant.
- Identify the behaviours that they carry out to avoid these situations (or what they find troublesome about them) and the

behaviours that they carry out when they are in these situations which may make their problems worse. Here, you will seek to help your clients to assess what happens in response to their behaviours.

- Identify how they 'feel like' acting in these situations but do not convert into overt behaviour.
- Identify the distorted and unrealistic thinking that accompany their troublesome emotion.
- Identify their rigid and extreme attitudes towards the adversity that account for their troublesome emotions, unconstructive behaviour and distorted/unrealistic thinking. These are their *B*asic attitudes.

Initially, you will show your clients how to use the assessment form in a therapy session using a recent problem episode. Here, initially, you will take the lead and guide your clients towards identifying the relevant information by asking them focused questions. You will then probably ask them to complete a new assessment form before the next therapy session on another specific problem episode and will go over their responses at the beginning of that session. You will then give your clients feedback to help them to use the form more accurately. This process will continue to the point where they can use the form on their own.

After they have become proficient at using the form, they hopefully will be able to carry out an assessment in their head by referring to its categories either before they encounter a relevant adversity or even while they are in the midst of experiencing one. If they need help to do this, provide them with such assistance.

Helping Your Clients Learn How to Examine Their Attitudes

Here, you help your client to learn how to examine the rigid and extreme attitudes that underpin their problems and the flexible and non-extreme alternative attitudes. In my view the best way you can help them to learn these skills of attitude examination is in a structured way.

Here is one way of doing this:

- Have them take their rigid attitude and the flexible attitude alternative.[1]
- While encouraging them to consider these attitudes together suggest that they ask and answer fully the following questions.
  - Which attitude is true and which is false and why?
  - Which attitude is logical and which is illogical and why?
  - Which attitude is helpful and which is unhelpful and why?
  - Which attitude would you teach your children and why?
- After the client has learned to do this on paper, encourage them to use this skill in their heads, first in imagery and then in actual situations.

While REBT largely focuses on helping clients to develop flexible and non-extreme attitudes, you will also want to teach your clients other skills either when they get stuck using attitude examination skills or after they have derived benefit from applying such skills.

Helping Your Clients Learn 'Acceptance-Based' Thinking Skills

Acceptance-based thinking skills are not generally taught by using written forms; rather they are taught experientially (i.e., by clients gaining experience in the use of such skills). Here, you may ask your clients to identify a meaningful metaphor which helps them to digest the idea that they can recognize the existence of a disturbed emotion or problematic form of thinking without engaging with it, on the one hand, and without trying to eliminate it, on the other. You will also introduce them to various exercises which will help them to develop these acceptance-based thinking skills and you will suggest that they practise these skills in relevant situations. How and at what rate you do this is a matter for negotiation between you and your clients. Finally, you will encourage your clients to practise these skills while pursuing value-based goals.

Helping Your Clients to Learn Behavioural Skills

Another area in which you can help your clients to become their own REBT therapist involves their acquiring key behavioural skills which will help them to achieve and maintain their goals. Commonly taught behavioural skills in REBT include communication, assertion and study skills.

Communication Skills

Here you help your clients learn, among others, how to:

- Listen actively to what others say.
- Convey their understanding of what these others are saying.
- State clearly what they want to say.

These skills are particularly important to developing and maintaining good relationships with others.

Assertion Skills

Here, you help clients to state clearly their position on various matters that serve to help them to maintain healthy boundaries between themselves and others. Assertion skills enable your clients (i) to convey their negative feelings to others while showing respect for them and, equally important, they also enable your clients (ii) to convey their positive feelings to these others. The skills in the first category are particularly relevant for those who often do what they don't want to do and therefore get taken advantage of in relationships, and the skills in the second category are more relevant for those who other people complain always focus on negative aspects of their relationships to the exclusion of the positive aspects.

Study Skills

Here you help clients learn, among others, how to:

- Organize what you have to do on a course of study.
- Digest information.
- Convey your ideas in writing to enable you to achieve your academic goals.

These are just a sample of behavioural skills that you can help your clients learn in REBT when they do not have such skills in their behavioural repertoire and where the acquisition of such skills is important in helping them to achieve and maintain their therapeutic goals.

The Process of Learning Behavioural Skills

While you will help your clients to learn and internalize the above-mentioned skills in ways that best suit their learning style, acquiring behavioural skills as part of your clients becoming their own REBT therapist is likely to involve some or all of the following steps:

- You will help your clients identify the relevant behavioural skill deficit and encourage them to see how learning this skill will help them to achieve their therapeutic goals and how doing so will stand them in good stead for the future. As part of this process you will encourage your clients to share any DROs to learning the skill which you will discuss with them in full.

- You will then outline the skill and break it down into its constituent parts and will model this skill for your clients if necessary and where practicable.
- Your clients will then try out the skill, first in the therapy session, if this can be done, and be encouraged to implement the skill in their own personal style.
- Then, you will encourage them to practise the skill before the next therapy session.
- They will report back on their experiences of implementing the skill and be given feedback on how to refine it.
- Through this process of skill practice and refinement, based on experience and feedback, your clients will internalize this skill and be able to use it in the future whenever they need to do so.
- During this process of behavioural skill learning and practice, your clients may encounter a variety of obstacles along the way. I refer you to Chapter 7, where I devoted an entire chapter to identifying and dealing with obstacles to making progress in REBT. I want to make the point here that you should encourage your clients to disclose such obstacles to skill learning and internalization to you so that together you may understand and respond effectively to the factors leading to the obstacle.

Helping Your Clients Learn Emotion Regulation Skills

A recent development in REBT and CBT has been the focus that therapists place on helping clients to regulate their distressed emotions so that they don't feel overwhelmed by them. Some of the skills that I have already discussed form a part of your clients learning to regulate their emotions. Thus, helping your clients to look for and respond to the attitudes that underpin their distressed emotions will generally help to abate them, as will externalizing them in some way, as it is often the act of suppressing these emotions that adds to your clients' distress. Also, suggesting to clients to communicate respectfully to another person how they feel helps in this regard, as does writing their feelings down. In addition, having clients learn and practise mindfulness-based skills, where they acknowledge the presence of their distressed emotion and continue to pursue their goals without engaging with the emotion or trying to eliminate it, often serves to reduce the subjective nature of their distress.

In addition to these methods, you may use some or all of the following to teach your clients how to regulate their distressing emotions.

Developing Unconditional Self-Acceptance

Your clients might find a negative emotion particularly distressing because they are judging themselves negatively for experiencing the emotion. The presence of shame for having a feeling is a good sign that they are doing this (e.g. regarding themselves as childish and less worthwhile for feeling hurt). Here, you will want to teach your clients to accept themselves as an ordinary person experiencing an understandable emotion and help them to see that judging themselves on the basis of an experience is neither valid nor helpful to them.

Learning Self-Validation and Self-Compassion

Self-validation occurs when your clients are able to reassure themselves that what they feel inside is real, is important and makes sense given the circumstances in which they felt it. Self-compassion extends this in three ways, as noted by the psychologist Dr Kristin Neff: (i) by encouraging your clients to relate to themselves with kindness, (ii) by encouraging your clients to see that they are not different from others but are part of common humanity, as we all struggle with distressing feelings at times, and (iii) by encouraging your clients to develop a mindful stance for their feelings (as noted above). Help your clients to take these concepts and to use them in everyday ways and suggest the same process of (i) practice, (ii) feedback and (iii) refinement that I discussed earlier in this chapter.

In my view, helping people to accept themselves is best done before encouraging them to use the skills of self-validation and self-compassion.

Increasing Distress Tolerance

One of the major reasons why your clients may find their emotions difficult to regulate is that their stance towards these emotions indicates that they find them intolerable. As a result, they may try to get rid of them or away from them as soon as they begin to experience them or they may attempt to avoid situations in which they predict that they might experience them. Some CBT therapists call this 'experiential avoidance', where your clients literally attempt to avoid experiencing certain emotions. In order to develop a sense of regulation over these emotions, you need to help your clients to increase their level of tolerance for these emotions. As they do so, they will become less fearful of their emotions and this will help them to deal with the issues that underpin them.

Using Imagery to Deal with Feelings

Approaches to REBT not only focus on thinking that occurs in words; they also focus on thinking that occurs in images. You should thus help your clients to use imagery by picturing themselves in troublesome situations and dealing constructively with the feelings that they predict they will experience.

Encouraging them to rehearse such scenarios will again help them to become less afraid of their feelings and to face them rather than avoid them.

Using Self-Soothing Skills

In the same way that a mother soothes her baby when the child is upset, you can encourage your clients to utilize their five senses to learn to soothe themselves as a means of regulating their distressing emotions.

Learning Relapse Prevention Skills

One very important way in which your clients can become their own therapist is by learning relapse prevention skills. These involve your helping them do the following:

- Accepting without liking the reality of lapses or slips (i.e. temporary and non-serious return to their problems).
- Identifying vulnerability factors (i.e. factors both in your clients' environment and within themselves that serve as triggers to lapses/slips).
- Developing and rehearsing constructive responses to these vulnerability factors.
- Facing up to these vulnerability factors in a sensible way so that they can practise these constructive responses.
- Accepting themselves if they relapse (i.e. a more serious and enduring return to their problems) and learning from this experience.

Helping Clients to Generalize Learning, to Become Less Prone to Emotional Disturbance in the Future and to Pursue Healthy Self-Development

Whether your clients have sought help from you for one problem or for several problems, you can give them the option to add to their skills as their own therapist once they have achieved what they were seeking from REBT. First, you can help them to generalize their learning; second, you can help them learn to become less prone to emotional disturbance in the future; and third, you can encourage them to pursue matters of healthy self-development.

Before I discuss these three issues, I want to make clear that addressing them in therapy is dependent on three points:

1. Whether or not your clients want to learn these skills.
2. Whether or not you as therapist conceive of working with these issues as being a part of your role.
3. Whether or not the context in which you are seeing your clients permits such work, given the amount of time that needs to be devoted to it.

As with other matters, you need to discuss such issues with your clients and come to an agreement with them on these issues. However, assuming that both of you want to and are able to focus on such issues and, if relevant, you have the support of the organization in which you seeing your clients, then the following points should be borne in mind.

Helping Clients to Generalize Learning

Once your clients have achieved their therapeutic goal, or one of them if they have several, then they have the option of generalizing the learning that they derived from achieving their goal(s) to tackling other problems that they may have. You can help your clients do this by working with them to identify what they learned, to see if this learning is appropriate to their other problems, and helping them to determine a plan based on their learning to tackle these problems, if relevant. Asking your clients the following questions may help you in your discussions with them on this point.

• What recurring attitudes, thoughts and images did you identify as being at the core of your problem(s), and how did you respond constructively to them? Are these attitudes, thoughts and images relevant to your other problems and, if so, would responding to them in a similar way also have a constructive impact as you deal with your new problems? If so, how can you best do so?

- What recurring behavioural patterns did you identify as being relevant in understanding how you unwittingly maintained your problems and what more constructive alternative behaviours did you implement in achieving your goals? Are these problematic behaviours also a factor in your other problems and, if so, can you apply the more constructive alternative behaviours that you developed in addressing your previous problems to these new problems?

Helping Clients to Become Less Prone to Emotional Disturbance in the Future

If your clients want to become less prone to emotional disturbance in the future, you need to help them learn and apply general patterns of flexible/non-extreme thinking and constructive behaviour to a range of adversities that are likely to be troublesome for them. Encouraging them to seek out such adversities, wherever possible and feasible, in a sensible way, while using these general patterns, is probably the best way of helping them to do this. This is best implemented when the task at hand is difficult but not overwhelming for your client. If you and your client have decided to work on helping them to become less prone to future emotional disturbance, the extent to which you agree on how you will approach this task is once again important.

Helping Clients to Pursue Healthy Self-Development

Your clients may have wondered about the difference between therapy and coaching. One way that I distinguish the two for them is that therapy is more concerned with helping them overcome emotional problems, whereas coaching is focused on helping them to pursue goals that are related to healthy self-development. While the differences are, in fact, more blurred than this in reality, it is a useful rule of thumb when considering the differences between REBT and Rational Emotive Behaviour Coaching (REBC) for present purposes. Thus, when you are predominantly working with your clients on matters largely concerned with promoting their healthy self-development, strictly speaking, you have moved into coaching and this needs to be acknowledged by both of you. Most organizations that offer non-fee-paying therapy do not regard coaching, by this definition, as part of their brief, and if your clients are paying you a fee and getting reimbursed from a private health organization, it is useful for you and your clients to be aware that it is unlikely that these organizations will pay for coaching as opposed to therapy. However, if you are seeing your clients privately, are not seeking fee reimbursement and have coaching as well as therapy skills, then REBC can be seen as a logical extension of successful REBT.

In the final chapter of this guide, I will discuss the situation where your client, at the outset, chooses to commit themself to only one session with you. You may think that there is little you can do in this situation. However, as I will show you, if you draw upon what is called the single-session mindset and upon an REBT-informed way of working with your client in this circumstance, then there is a lot you can do.

Note

1   This schema can also be used with the client's main extreme and non-extreme attitude.

Chapter 9

When a Client Only Commits to One Session

This Therapist Guide is based on what I call the conventional therapy mindset. This way of thinking about therapy sees the practice of therapy as stretching out over time with a beginning, a middle and an end, usually lasting for a good number of sessions. This is how REBT therapists have been trained in its practice and it is the dominant viewpoint in our field. A good friend and colleague of mine, Dr Michler Bishop, who was trained in REBT, once said that the purpose of the first session of psychotherapy was to ensure that the client came back for the second session.

However, if one considers the attendance data at psychotherapy clinics across the world, one finds an interesting fact. That is that the modal[1] number of sessions that clients have at these clinics is one, followed by two, followed by three, etc. When people learn about this finding they immediately think that clients who attend one session of therapy must have been dissatisfied with the session and decided not to return. However, the picture is very different. About 70%–80% of those who have one session are satisfied with that session. Furthermore, when clinics are organized such that incoming clients all have a single session of therapy on entry rather than an assessment session, then 50% of those clients decide that they got what they wanted from the session and don't request any further sessions.

The implication of these findings is that you, as an REBT therapist, need to be prepared to offer help to clients who choose, for a number of reasons, to attend for only one session of REBT. What might these reasons be?

DOI: 10.4324/9781003493150-10

First, the client may have a problem for which they are seeking help and they think that they can be helped with that problem in one session. They may have sought help from you because they know that you are an REBT therapist and think that REBT can be helpful to them. On the other hand, they may know nothing about REBT, but think that one focused session with a therapist is all they need and are looking for.

Second, the client wants a single session with you, as an REBT therapist, not because they expect such a session to be all the help they need but because they want guidance from you concerning how they can tackle their nominated problem independently going forward. When I have an injury and seek help from a physiotherapist, I want that person to teach me what to do so I can practise these techniques on my own. I don't want to keep coming back to rehearse the techniques in the presence of the practitioner.

Third, the client may seek a single session of REBT to discover whether this approach to therapy is right for them or not. Effectively, they are taking REBT for a test drive!

Finally, the client may come for a single session seeking signposting help from you concerning whether or not REBT will suit them and, if not, what therapeutic approach will suit them better. This group of clients do not expect their contact with you to provide a solution to their problem in the session itself, but they want a pathway that they can follow where they can address their problems over time with a therapy or therapist that is right for them. They want you to help them make that decision. This may be with you as their REBT therapist or, as noted above, it may be with a therapist who practises differently from you.

The George Kelly Dictum

The above single-session therapy scenarios and the more conventional therapy scenario raise the question concerning how you are to know what the client is looking for when they contact you. Extrapolating from a well-known quotation of George Kelly, the originator of Personal Construct Psychology, 'If you want to know what help the client wants, ask them – they may tell you'.[2]

Therefore, once a prospective client contacts you, then one way to respond is to discover what help they are looking for by directly asking them as shown in the next section.

Ask the Client What Help They Are Looking For

Here is an example of what you can say to a client who first approaches you as a prospective client. It shows how this question is influenced by adopting a single-session mindset.

Thank you for contacting me. I would like to find out from you what help you are looking for, so let me outline the possibilities as I see them.

1. You may be looking for ongoing therapy for a number of issues that you want to address and would like me to help you in this regard.
2. You may have one or two issues that you want to address and are happy to do so in brief therapy (e.g., six sessions, spread out by negotiation).
3. You have one issue that you want to address and are hopeful that I can help you do that in one visit. At the end of the session, you will be clearer if we have done that or if you need another session or more sessions.
4. You have a number of issues and are interested in learning how REBT might be helpful to you. While you think that you will need more help than one session, you are hopeful that I will (a) outline how you can use REBT independently to do the work yourself and (b) suggest some materials to aid you in this regard.

5. You want one session to discuss what type of help may be most helpful to you going forward. You would like me to signpost you to the most suitable form of help.

I would be interested to get your thoughts about these possibilities.

In the rest of this chapter, I will discuss the scenario where the person is seeking a single session to be helped with a specific issue.

When the Client Wants a Single Session

When a client indicates that they want you to help them in a single session and you feel able to comply with that request, you need to help them in the following ways. What follows shows how you can use practical suggestions from adopting a single-session therapy (SST) mindset and from REBT.

If Possible, Send the Client a Pre-Session Form to Complete and Return

If you have the opportunity to do so, it is a good idea to ask the client to prepare for the session. The more preparatory work they can do before they see you, the clearer they are likely to be on what they want to focus on in the session and to take away from it. However, do not make it mandatory for them to complete the pre-session form. Rather, invite them to do so and also invite them to return it to you before the session so that you can also prepare for the session. See Appendix 4 for an example of such a form.

Get the Client's Informed Consent for Single-Session Therapy

As with other modes of helping, it is important that the client gives their informed consent for single-session therapy. To do that, they first need to be informed about what SST is. In my view, SST is 'a purposeful endeavour where both parties set out with the intention of helping the client in one session knowing that more help is available, if needed'. After informing the client of this, answer any questions that they may have until they are happy to give their consent.

It is also useful to get the client's permission for you to refer to their completed pre-session form since doing so will not only save time but help you with your interventions.

At the Outset, Ask the Client to Nominate a Problem and Agree a Focus

Most people seeking single-session therapy will be looking for help to solve a specific problem, although this is not universally the case. Sometimes, the person may be looking to understand their problem better, for example. However, it is still worth asking a question such as, 'And if you understood the issue better, what do you hope such understanding would lead to?' This is because some clients do say that they hope understanding would lead to problem solution.

Given that most clients are looking for help with a specific problem with which they have become stuck, it is important to agree with them which problem you are going to focus on (I call this the 'nominated problem'). This is important since sometimes clients come with more than one problem they want help with.

Interrupt the Client, if Necessary

Once you have agreed on a focus for the session (this will be the client's nominated problem) and you start to work on the problem with your client, be aware that you may need to interrupt them to retain the agreed focus. Given this, before you start work on their nominated problem, it is useful to give the client a rationale for interrupting them, if necessary. Here is what I say to my SST clients on this point:

> Sometimes, I may need to interrupt you in order to keep us focused on the problem you want help with. This is because we may wander away from the focus, and it is important that I bring us back to it. May I have your permission to do this?

Once the client has given their permission for me to interrupt them, I will ask them how I can best do so and then implement their chosen method if and when the need arises.

Negotiate the Client's Goal for the Session and for Their Nominated Problem

It is difficult to do effective single-session therapy work if you and your client are not doing purposive work. This means agreeing goals with your client. There are two sets of goals that are important to consider in REBT-informed single-session therapy: session goals and problem-related goals

Session Goals

A session goal represents what the client wants and can realistically be expected to take away from the session that is relevant to their nominated problem. This is quite often a solution which they need to implement after the session in order to address the nominated problem.

Problem-Related Goals

A problem-related goal is what the person seeks to achieve in relation to the nominated problem so that the problem has been rendered a non-problem. As mentioned above, the client

```
Nominated Problem ------------→ Session Goal   -----------→ Problem-Related Goal
                                    |                              ∧
                                    |                              |
                                    |                              |
                                    |                              |
                                 Solution  -------------------→ After the Session
```

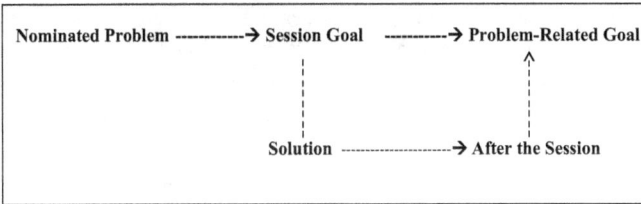

Figure 9.1 The Relationship between the Nominated Problem, and Session-Related and Problem-Related Goals

Note: This figure shows that a session goal is often a solution to the nominated problem that the client needs to implement after the session so that they can achieve their problem-related goal.

needs to implement the selected solution and do so over time to achieve their problem-related goal.

Figure 9.1 outlines the relationship between the client's nominated problem and their session-related and problem-related goals.

Check That the Client Is Still Talking about What Is Important to Them

While keeping to the agreed focus is important in SST, you need to check periodically that your client is still discussing an issue that is important to them. If not, and you have time, then it is important to change tack to what is more important to the client. However, if you have taken time and care to help the client select their nominated problem, then this shift is unlikely to occur.

Discover How the Client Has Attempted to Solve the Problem Before

Before introducing REBT to the client to show them what it has to offer them as they strive to find a solution to their problem, it is important for you to discover what the client has previously tried to solve the problem. People frequently try a variety of strategies to help themselves well before they reach out to seek professional help. While none of these strategies will have proven completely successful – for if they had, the client would not be seeking therapeutic help – some of what they have tried before may have had some value and can contribute towards the construction of a solution now.

Also, it is useful for you to discover what the client has tried in the past that hasn't proven helpful to them – or even led to a deterioration of their problem – so you can rule out potential solutions that haven't helped the client.

Discover Successful Strategies That the Client Has Used with Other Problems

It is also useful to discover if the client has solved other emotionally related problems that may be different to their current nominated problem. Helping the client to see that they can apply strategies that have proven successful for them in other spheres to their current nominated problem is often quite fruitful.

Identify and Utilize the Client's Internal and External Resources

The single-session mindset encourages you to look actively for both the client's internal and external resources so that you can help the client to make use of them at salient times during the session and afterwards.

Identify and Utilize the Client's Internal Resources

With respect to internal resources, these tend to be tender-minded (e.g., compassion, empathy, kindness) or tough-minded (e.g., resilience, grit, assertion) and they can be obtained directly (e.g., 'Which strengths do you have as a person that might help you in our work together on your nominated problem?') or discerned indirectly (e.g., 'Listening to you talk, it strikes me how resilient you have been in putting up with this situation for so long'). The client can draw on their internal resources in developing a solution to their problem in the session or in applying the solution after the session.

Identify and Utilize the Client's External Resources

A client's external resources may include (i) people in their lives who can encourage them in their efforts to implement their selected solution, (ii) organizations that may offer support and (iii) materials (e.g., therapeutic/educational that may aid them in solution implementation).

Offer the REBT Perspective on Their Problem and Its Solution

Some clients will not require any input from REBT to achieve their session goals. In such cases, the two of you can devise a solution that stems from the issues you have covered and this can be done without reference to REBT. Other clients do seem to require additional input in that what you have discussed with them has not yielded potential solutions. In these cases, I suggest that you ask your client a question such as, 'Are you interested in my take on what we have discussed so far?' When the client says that they are interested then you can offer your REBT-informed view of their problems and how they can best deal with it. Of course, when the client has approached you for single-session help precisely because you are an REBT therapist, then you can use REBT from the outset together with the more general issues that I have discussed so far. I will discuss now discuss how you can efficiently use REBT within a single-session format.

Assess the Problem Using the **ABC** Framework

When the client nominates a problem to discuss in the single session, it is good REBT practice for you to encourage them to select a specific example of this problem for you to assess. A specific example means that the problem-related episode took place in a concrete situation with particular people present acting in identifiable ways. Such a specific example of the problem can be a recent example, a vivid example, a typical example or an anticipated example. The advantage of selecting an anticipated example is that once the example has been assessed and a solution developed then the client can implement this solution in a similar future situation.

In using the *ABC* framework to assess the client's selected example, the most common order is *CAB*. You begin by identifying the most problematic unhealthy negative emotion (UNE) at *C* experienced by the client in the situation, together with its major behavioural and thinking concomitants. Once you have identified the major UNE, you use it to find the aspect of the situation that the client was most disturbed about. This is the adversity at *A*. The most efficient way of doing this, in my view, is to use a technique called 'Windy's Magic Question' or WMQ (see Appendix 5).

Then, when you have assessed both *C* and *A*, you can use the information you have gleaned so far to identify the client's rigid/ extreme attitude and corresponding flexible/non-extreme attitude at *B*. Again, in my opinion, the most efficient way of doing this is to use a technique called 'Windy's Review Assessment Procedure' or WRAP (see Appendix 6).

Promote Intellectual Insight: Help the Client to Examine Their Attitudes

The heart of REBT is attitude change. This is the solution that REBT offers the client in single-session work. There are two phases of such change: intellectual insight and emotional insight[3] (see Chapter 7). Intellectual insight, in this context, is achieved when the client understands lightly and occasionally that their rigid and extreme attitudes are false, illogical and yield largely unconstructive results for them and that their alternative flexible and non-extreme attitudes are true, logical and yield largely constructive results for them. Intellectual insight is not sufficient for attitude change. Thus, it provides knowledge but does not impact significantly on the client's feelings and behaviour. Clients with intellectual insight say such things as 'I understand it in my head but don't feel it in my gut'. However, intellectual insight is necessary for clients to have and the most efficient way of promoting such insight is to use what I call the 'Choice-Based Examination Method' (see Appendix 7).

Promote Emotional Insight: Putting Intellectual Insight into Practice

By contrast, emotional insight, in this context, is achieved when the client has a deeply held conviction that their rigid and extreme attitudes are false, illogical and yield largely unconstructive results for them and that their alternative flexible and non-extreme attitudes are true, logical and yield largely constructive results for them. Emotional insight is a sign that attitude change is underway. As such, having emotional insight does impact significantly on the client's feelings and behaviour. Clients with emotional insight say such things as 'Not only do I understand it in my head, I also feel it in my gut'.

The best way that you can help the client implement the attitude change solution that they have selected is to help them to put their intellectual insight into practice until it becomes emotional insight. This is done in the first instance by you developing an action plan with your client.

Help the Client to Develop an Action Plan and Get Their Commitment to Implement It[4]

The purpose of an action plan from an REBT perspective is to encourage the client to take action in the face of their problem-related adversity that is consistent with their newly chosen flexible/non-extreme attitude and inconsistent with their currently held rigid/extreme attitude.

Elements of a Good Action Plan

As such, it should be remembered that results from a single session are achieved by what your client does outside the session. Also, the achievement of the client's session goal represents the beginning of a process of change rather than the end of it, namely when the client has reached their problem-related goal. Having made this point, let me discuss several features of a good action plan that should be considered by both you and your client as you work together to draw up such a plan.

CLIENT RESPONSIBILITY

The client needs to take responsibility for implementing the plan. If the client is not prepared to take ownership of implementing the action plan, then there is no point in the therapist helping them to develop the plan. Thus, before such work is undertaken the therapist should ascertain that the client is prepared to do whatever they agree should be a part of the action plan.

INTEGRATING THE SOLUTION INTO THE CLIENT'S LIFE

The client should be able to integrate the plan into their life. If they are not able to do this, they may begin to initiate the plan but quickly stop doing so because the effort required is, in their mind, too great. I am not suggesting here that the client should only implement an action when it is easy for them to do so. What I am saying is that when it is part of the client's everyday routine, then they are more likely to implement the plan over time than when it is not part of their schedule. For example, it is not easy for a person with diabetes to inject themself with insulin several times a day but if they make it part of their daily routine then they will be able to maintain doing so.

THE IMPORTANCE OF CLARITY

What the client has agreed to do in the action plan needs to be clear. Therefore, the more specific the solution that is delineated in the plan, the better.

REMEMBERING THE PURPOSE OF THE SOLUTION

The client needs to see clearly how implementing the action plan can lead to the achievement of their problem-related goal. It will also help if the client keeps this connection at the forefront of their mind when implementing the solution in their everyday life.

The Components of a Good Action Plan

Perhaps the most important part of a solution-focused action plan is its components. These components are as follows:

- *What* the client has agreed to do (i.e., the aspects of the solution).
- *When* the client has agreed to implement the solution.
- *Where* the solution is to be implemented.
- *Whom* the solution is to be implemented with.
- *How often* is the solution to be implemented.

Get the Client's Commitment to Implement the Action Plan

A commitment is a firm promise that your client makes with themself to implement the action plan. It is *not* a commitment made to you and, as such, you need to take yourself out of the equation. It may be that your client has a doubt, reservation or objection to making the commitment with themself and it is important that you ask them to ask themself if they have such a DRO. If they say 'no' to this question, I suggest that you follow up with this question: 'If you had such a doubt, reservation or objection to making a firm promise with yourself to carry out the action plan, what would it be?' Sometimes asking this supplementary question gives the client permission to disclose such a DRO which you can then discuss with them. The purpose of this discussion is to help the person clear the path to making a commitment with themself to implement their action plan.

IDENTIFYING AND DEALING WITH ANTICIPATED OBSTACLES

In addition to dealing with any DROs your client may have about committing themself to implementing the action plan, it is also very useful for you to help them to identify potential obstacles to them carrying it out. This is to help them to think about how they would respond should they encounter any obstacles that they anticipate.

MAKING A COMMITMENT PUBLIC OR KEEPING IT PRIVATE

When discussing making a commitment to implementing the action plan, it is useful to discover if your client finds value in making their commitment public or keeping it private. By making their commitment public either generally or to certain people (e.g., those whom they regard as being among their external resources), some clients experience a strengthened sense of resolve, which will help them implement their action plan. Other clients prefer to keep their commitment private. With those clients, it is worthwhile discussing the advantages and disadvantages of making their commitment part of a written contract with themselves.

Ending the Session Well

Once you have helped the client to make a commitment to implementing their agreed action plan, this is a reliable sign that the session is coming to an end. When this happens, I suggest that you ask the client to summarize the session.

Ask the Client for a Summary of the Session

There are two main reasons why it is better to ask the client to summarize the session rather than providing your own summary. The first reason is that it keeps the client actively involved in the session and encourages them to use their brain to summarize rather than borrow your brain for the purpose. The second reason is that the client is more likely to take away what they regard as important from the session than what you regard to be important. Thus, asking the client to provide their own summary encourages them to think about what for them were the highlights of the session. On the other hand, your summary would focus on what were the highlights for you.

Ideally, the client's summary should include the nature of the nominated problem the two of you discussed, the solution you came up with to address the problem, and the action plan you agreed which the client has given their commitment to implement.

Elicit the Client's Takeaways

In SST, a client's takeaway is what the client has learned from the session that, in their mind, is worth taking away from the session. This may be covered in the client's summary, or the client may disclose it once you have asked for it. It is important that you do not overload the client at this point. One or two takeaways deemed important by the client, which they think will make a significant difference to their life going forward, are better than several that emanate from you that may confuse or overwhelm the client.

Ideally, then, the client should leave the session with a solution, an action plan and new learning derived from their conversation with you.

Encourage the Client to Generalize the Solution and/or Their Takeaways

If feasible, you should ask the client if they can see ways of generalizing (a) the solution that you have helped them to develop and (b) their takeaways to other relevant aspects of their life that you haven't discussed with them. For example, if you have helped the client to develop a good solution to dealing with criticism at work, ask them if they can use the solution in other settings where they may face criticism. Also, ask them if what they have learned is applicable to other adversities that they struggle with that they have not had an opportunity to discuss with you.

In general, most clients need help to generalize what they learn from therapy sessions and if you do not provide them with such an opportunity, they may not think of doing so themselves.

Provide a Final Opportunity for Comments or Questions

Given that you want to end the session well, it is important to give your client a last opportunity of to tell you something that they would regret not telling you or asking you something that they would regret not asking. In giving them this final chance, it is important that you make clear that it needs to be relevant to what you covered with them in the session. It should not be viewed as an invitation to bring up a new problem in the closing moments of the session.

Agree the Way Forward

You will recall from my definition of single-session therapy, that having the session does not preclude the client from accessing further help. Having said this, SST does provide an opportunity for clients to leave the session with what they have come for. Most SST practitioners consider that it is important for clients to have an opportunity to reflect on what they have learned, digest their learning and implement their action plan to see how they get on before making a decision concerning whether or not to seek further help. Thus, it is not a good idea in general to offer the client an opportunity at the end of the session to make an appointment for a further session. There will, of course, be exceptions to this. Thus, what your client has discussed with you may have evoked strong feelings that have not been resolved at the end of the session and you both consider that harm would befall the client if a further session is not arranged before the client leaves.

However, it is generally a good idea to give your client an opportunity to get the most from the session and this is done by giving them time to put into practice what they have learned from the session and to see what happens. At that point, they may decide they don't need further help or they may decide that they do. The choice is up to them.

We have now come to the end of this Therapist Guide and I hope you have found it useful and that it has given you some ideas concerning how to help your clients to get the most out of REBT. I would appreciate receiving any feedback that might improve this guide based on your experiences of using it. Please email me at windy@windydryden.com

Notes

1 The mode is the most frequently occurring number in a series of numbers.
2 Kelly's actual quotation was, 'If you want to know what's wrong with someone, ask them – they may tell you!'
3 I will discuss emotional insight below.
4 This section is relevant whether you have helped the client to select an REBT-informed solution or one not informed by REBT.

What Is Rational Emotive Behaviour Therapy?

There are a number of approaches to therapy and it is important that you understand something of the one that I practise which is known as Rational Emotive Behaviour Therapy (REBT). REBT is based on an old idea attributed to Epictetus, a Roman philosopher, who said that 'Men are disturbed not by things, but by their views of things'. In REBT, we have modified this and say: 'People are not disturbed by the adversities that they face. Rather, they disturb themselves about these adversities by the rigid and extreme attitudes that they hold towards them.' Once they have disturbed themselves they try to get rid of their disturbed feelings in ways that ultimately serve to maintain their problems.

As an REBT therapist I will help you to identify, examine and change the rigid and extreme attitudes that we argue underpin your emotional problems and to develop alternative flexible and non-extreme attitudes. I will also help you to examine the ways in which you have tried to help yourself that haven't worked and encourage you to develop and practise more effective, longer-lasting strategies. At the beginning of therapy, we will consider your problems one at a time and I will teach you a framework which will help you to break down your problems into their constituent parts. I will also teach you a variety of methods for examining and changing your rigid and extreme attitudes and a variety of methods to help you to consolidate and strengthen your alternative flexible and non-extreme attitudes. As therapy proceeds, I will help you to take increasing responsibility for using these methods and my ultimate aim is to help you to become your own therapist. As this happens, we will meet less frequently until you feel you can cope on your own.

Therapeutic Contract with Windy Dryden

1. Length of therapy sessions

   Therapy sessions are 50 minutes in length unless otherwise agreed. They will be face-to-face or by Zoom. If the latter, I will provide you with a link the day before the session.

2. Fee

   My fee is £... per session pro rata. The method of payment is by mutual agreement. I will give you two months' notice of any increase to my fee.

   Please note that as your contract is with me, I expect you to pay me directly. I do not invoice insurance companies, but will provide you with receipts for you to claim reimbursement from them.

3. Cancellation policy

   My cancellation policy is as follows. In order for you to cancel a session without charge you need to give me 48 hours' notice. My full fee will be levied if notice within this period is not given. An exception to this is if you, or a member of your immediate family, suffer a sudden serious illness.

   If I cancel a session, I will give you 48 hours' notice. If I do not do so, then your next therapy session will be free of charge. An exception to this is if I, or a member of my immediate family, suffer a sudden serious illness.

4. Confidentiality policy

   My confidentiality policy is as follows. All sessions are confidential with the following exceptions:

- If you pose a serious threat to your own life or well-being and are not prepared to take steps to protect yourself, I will take steps to provide such protection.
- If you pose a serious threat to the life or well-being of another person and are not prepared to take steps to protect them, I will take steps to provide such protection.
- If I am legally mandated to make my notes available.
- If my fees are not paid and I take legal recourse to recover these fees.
- If you wish me to provide information about our sessions to a third party, I require notification of this request in writing.

5. My working environment
   - As I do not have waiting room facilities, I would be grateful if you would ring my bell at your appointed appointment time and not before.
   - Please do not attend a therapy session if you are intoxicated or are under the influence of a mind-altering drug.
   - Also, as the smell of cigarette smoke lingers and may affect other clients whom I may see after your session, I respectfully request that you do not smoke an hour before your session.
   - If we are meeting by Zoom, please ensure that you are on your own in a professional working space with good Wi-Fi.

I have read, understood and agree with the above points.

Signature of client.............. Signature of therapist.................

Print name......................... Print name ....

Date................................ Date ....

Possible Reasons for Not Completing Homework (Self-Help) Tasks

Name.............. Date..........

The following is a list of reasons that various clients have given for not doing their homework (self-help) tasks during the course of REBT. Because the speed of improvement depends primarily on the number of such tasks that you are willing to do, it is of great importance to pinpoint any reasons that you may have for not doing this work. It is important to look for these reasons at the time that you feel a reluctance to do your task or a desire to put off doing it. Hence, it is best to fill out this questionnaire at that time. If you have any difficulty filling out this form and returning it to your therapist, it might be best to do it together during a therapy session.

Rate each statement by ringing 'T' (True) or 'F' (False). 'T' indicates that you agree with it; 'F' means the statement does not apply at this time.

1. It seems that nothing can help me, so there is no point in trying.   T/F
2. It wasn't clear, I didn't understand what I had to do.   T/F
3. I thought that the particular method my therapist had suggested would not be helpful. I didn't really see the value of it.   T/F
4. It seemed too hard.   T/F
5. I am willing to do self-help tasks, but I keep forgetting.   T/F

6. I did not have enough time. I was too busy.   T/F
7. If I do something my therapist suggests I do, it's not
   as good as if I come up with my own ideas.   T/F
8. I don't really believe I can do anything to help
   myself.   T/F
9. I have the impression my therapist is trying to
   boss me around or control me.   T/F
10. I worry about my therapist's disapproval. I believe
    that what I do just won't be good enough for them.   T/F
11. I felt too bad, sad, nervous, upset (underline the
    appropriate word[s]) to do it.   T/F
12. It would have upset me to do the homework.   T/F
13. It was too much to do.   T/F
14. It's too much like going back to school again.   T/F
15. It seemed to be mainly for my therapist's benefit.   T/F
16. Homework or self-help tasks have no place
    in therapy.   T/F
17. Because of the progress I've made, these tasks
    are likely to be of no further benefit to me.   T/F
18. Because these tasks have not been helpful in the
    past, I couldn't see the point of doing this one.   T/F
19. I don't agree with this particular approach
    to therapy.   T/F
20. OTHER REASONS (please write them):

Pre-Session Form

I invite you to fill in this form before your session with me. This will help you to prepare for the session so that you can get the most from it. It also helps me to help you as effectively as I can. Please return it by email attachment before our session. Be brief and concise in your answers.

1. **What is the issue that you want to focus on in the session?**
   Be concise. In one or two sentences get to the heart of the problem, if possible.

2. **Why is this significant?**
   What's at stake? How does this affect your life? What is the future impact if the issue is not resolved?

3. **What is your goal in discussing this issue in the session?**
   What are the specific results you would like to achieve by the end of the session that would give you the sense that you have begun to make progress on the issue?

4. **Specify briefly the relevant background information.**
   What do you think I need to know about the issue to help you with it? Summarize in bullet points.

5. **How have you tried to deal with the issue up to this point?**
   What steps, successful or unsuccessful, have you taken so far in addressing the issue?

6. **What are the strengths or inner resources that you have as a person that you could draw upon while tackling the issue?**
   If you struggle with answering this question, think of what people who really know you and who are on your side would say.

7. **Who are the people in your life who can support you as you tackle the issue?**
   Name them and say what help each can provide.

8. **What help do you hope I can best provide you in the session? Please check the main <u>one</u>. Do not check more than one box.**
   - ☐ Help me to develop greater understanding of the issue
   - ☐ Help me by just listening while I talk about the issue
   - ☐ Help me to express my feelings about the issue
   - ☐ Help me to solve an emotional or behavioural problem; help me get unstuck
   - ☐ Help me to make a decision
   - ☐ Help me to resolve a dilemma
   - ☐ Help me by signposting me to the most appropriate service for my situation
   - ☐ Other (please specify):

Appendix 5

Windy's Magic Question

Purpose: To help the client to identify the *A* in the *ABC* framework as quickly as possible (i.e. what the client is most disturbed about) once *C* has been assessed and the situation in which *C* has occurred has been identified and briefly described.

Step 1: Have the client focus on their disturbed *C* (e.g. 'anxiety').

Step 2: Encourage the client to focus on the situation in which *C* occurred (e.g. 'about to give a public presentation to a group of consultants').

Step 3: Ask the client: *'Which ingredient could we give you to eliminate or significantly reduce C'* (here, anxiety)? (In this case the client said: 'my mind not going blank'). Take care that the client does not change the situation (i.e. they do not say: 'not giving the presentation').

Step 4: The opposite is probably *A* (e.g. 'my mind going blank'), but check. Ask: *'So when you were about to give the presentation, were you most anxious about your mind going blank'?* If not, use the question again until the client confirms what they were most anxious about in the described situation.

Windy's Review Assessment Procedure

[This follows on from Windy's Magic Question]

Purpose: Once C (e.g. 'anxiety') and A (e.g. 'my mind going blank') have been assessed, this technique can be used to identify both the client's rigid and alterative flexible attitude and to help the client to understand the two relevant B–C connections. This technique can also be used with any of the derivatives of the rigid and flexible attitude pairing

1. Begin by saying: *'Let's review what we know and what we don't know so far.'*
2. Then, say: *'We know three things.*
   First, we know that you were anxious (C).
   Second, we know that you were anxious about your mind going blank (A).
   Third, and this is an educated guess on my part, we know that it is important to you that your mind does not go blank. Am I correct?'
   Assuming that the client confirms your hunch, note that what you have done is to identify the part of the attitude that is common to both the client's rigid attitude and alternative flexible attitude, as we will see.
3. Continue by saying: *'Now let's review what we don't know. This is where I need your help. We don't know which of two attitudes your anxiety was based on. So, when you were anxious about your mind going blank, was your anxiety based on*

> *Attitude 1: "It is important to me that my mind does not go blank and therefore it must not do so" ("Rigid attitude") or*
>
> *Attitude 2: "It is important to me that my mind does not go blank, but that does not mean that it must not do so" ("Flexible attitude")?'*

4. If necessary, help the client to understand that their anxiety was based on their rigid attitude if they are unsure.

5. Once the client is clear that their anxiety was based on their rigid attitude, make and emphasize the rigid attitude– disturbed *C* connection. Then, ask: *'Now let's suppose instead that you had a strong conviction in attitude 2, how would you feel about your mind going blank if you strongly believed that while it was important to you that your mind did not go blank, it did not follow that it must not do so?'*

6. If necessary, help the client to nominate a healthy negative emotion such as concern, if not immediately volunteered, and make and emphasize the flexible attitude–healthy *C* connection.

7. Ensure that the client clearly understands the differences between the two *B–C* connections.

8. Encourage the client to set concern as the emotional goal in this situation and to see that developing conviction in their flexible attitude is the best way of achieving this goal.

Appendix 7

The Choice-Based Examination Method

[This follows on from Windy's Review Assessment Procedure]

Purpose: Once the client has understood the two B–C connections as outlined in the WRAP technique, the purpose of the Choice-Based Examination Method is to take their rigid and flexible attitudes together and to examine them with the goal of having the client choose which attitude they want to take forward. This method can also be used with any of the derivatives of the rigid and flexible attitude pairing.

Using the Choice-Based Examination Method with Rigid and Flexible Attitudes

1. When using this method with your client's rigid and flexible attitudes, first encourage them to focus on both attitudes.

Rigid Attitude	Flexible Attitude
'It is important to me that my mind does not go blank and therefore it must not do so'	'It is important to me that my mind does not go blank, but that does not mean that it must not do so'

2. Then, ask them the following questions:
   • Which of these two attitudes is true or consistent with reality and which is false or inconsistent with reality and why?

- Which of these two attitudes is logical or sensible and which is illogical or nonsensical and why?
- Which of these two attitudes is largely helpful to you and which is largely unhelpful to you and why?
- Which of these two attitudes would you teach to a group of children that you cared about and why?
- Which of these attitudes do you want to choose to develop going forward and why?

Using the Choice-Based Examination Method with Extreme and Non-Extreme Attitudes[1]

1. When using this method with your client's extreme and non-extreme attitudes, first encourage them to focus on both attitudes.

Extreme Attitude (e.g., Self-Devaluation Attitude)	Non-Extreme Attitude (e.g., Unconditional Self-Acceptance Attitude)
'It is bad if my mind goes blank and it would prove that I am a failure.'	'It is bad if my mind goes blank, but it would not prove that I am a failure. It would prove that I am a complex, fallible human being who can succeed and fail.'

2. Then, ask them the following questions:
   - Which of these two attitudes is true or consistent with reality and which is false or inconsistent with reality and why?
   - Which of these two attitudes is logical or sensible and which is illogical or nonsensical and why?

- Which of these two attitudes is largely helpful to you and which is largely unhelpful to you and why?
- Which of these two attitudes would you teach to a group of children that you cared about and why?
- Which of these attitudes do you want to choose to develop going forward and why?

Note

1   Here, the selected example of an extreme vs non-extreme attitude is the client's self-devaluation attitude vs their unconditional self-acceptance attitude. The same procedure is employed with the awfulizing vs non-awfulizing attitude pairing and the attitude of unbearability vs the attitude of unbearability pairing.

Index

For Product Safety Concerns and Information please contact our EU
representative GPSR@taylorandfrancis.com
Taylor & Francis Verlag GmbH, Kaufingerstraße 24, 80331 München, Germany

www.ingramcontent.com/pod-product-compliance
Lightning Source LLC
Chambersburg PA
CBHW052012270326
41929CB00015B/2892